Poppy

the YOGA Dog
A Kid's Guide to Stretch & Relax

Julianne Ososke

Published by Ososke Press
PO Box 1404 Mill Valley, CA 94942
United States of America

www.ososkepress.com

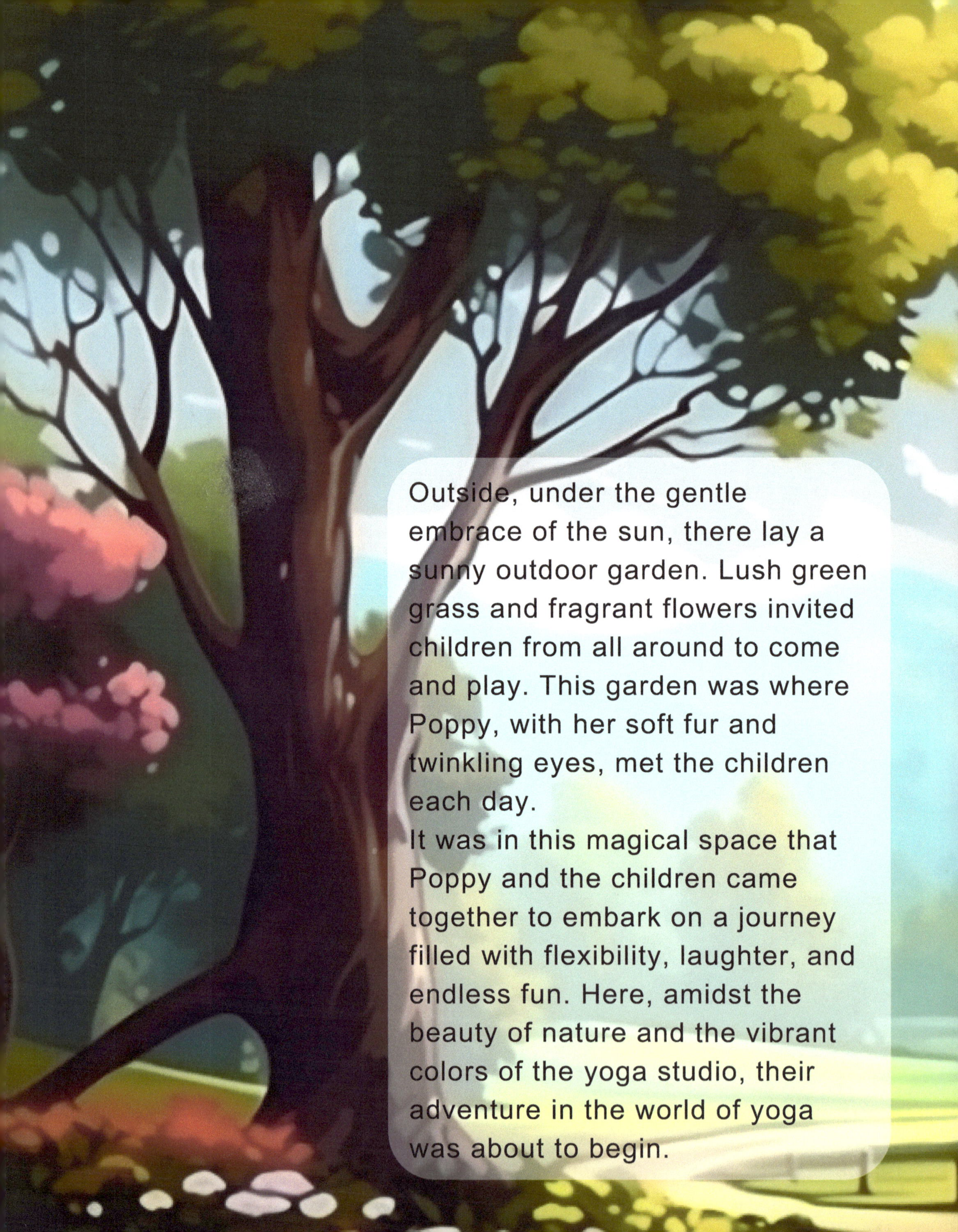

Outside, under the gentle embrace of the sun, there lay a sunny outdoor garden. Lush green grass and fragrant flowers invited children from all around to come and play. This garden was where Poppy, with her soft fur and twinkling eyes, met the children each day.

It was in this magical space that Poppy and the children came together to embark on a journey filled with flexibility, laughter, and endless fun. Here, amidst the beauty of nature and the vibrant colors of the yoga studio, their adventure in the world of yoga was about to begin.

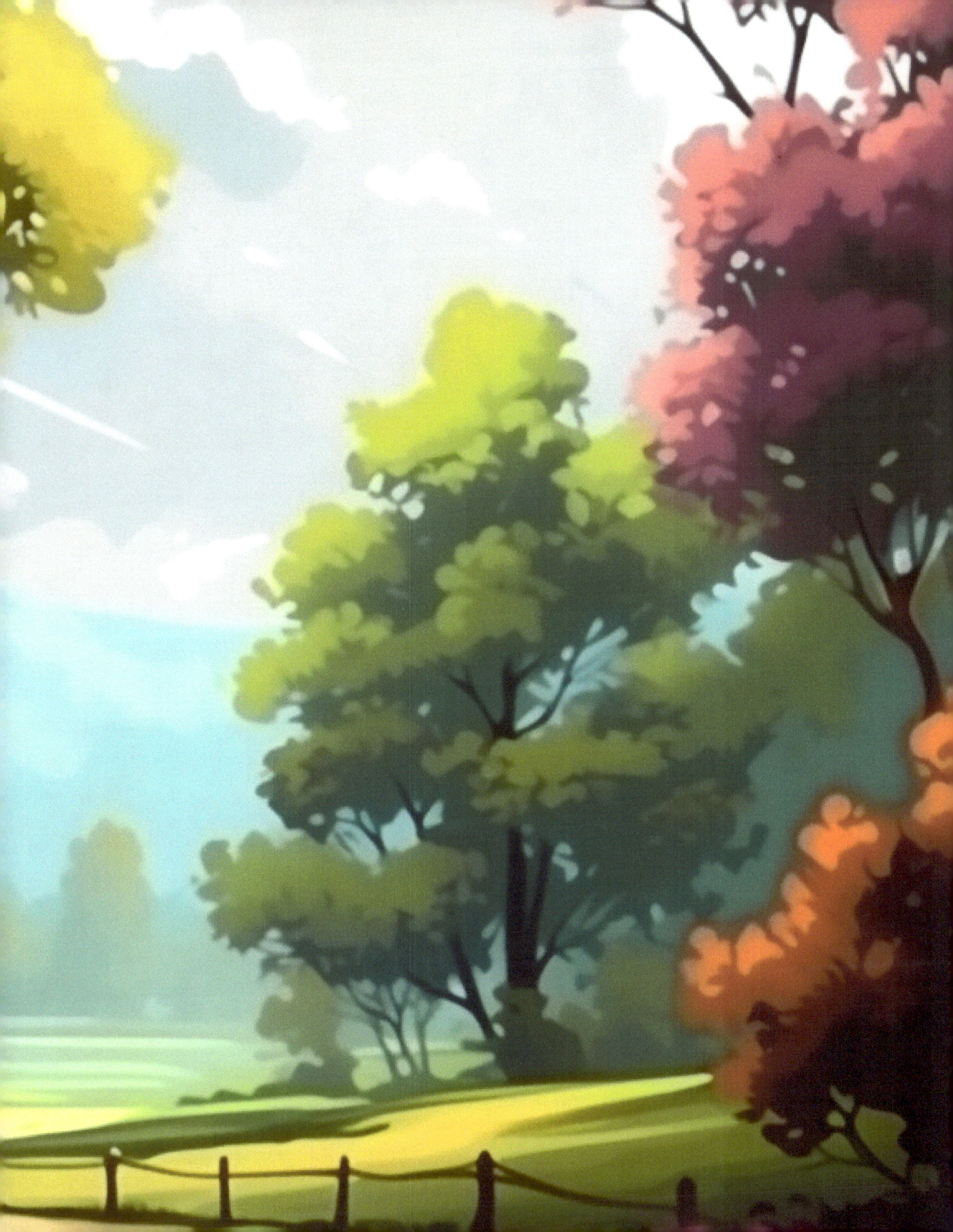

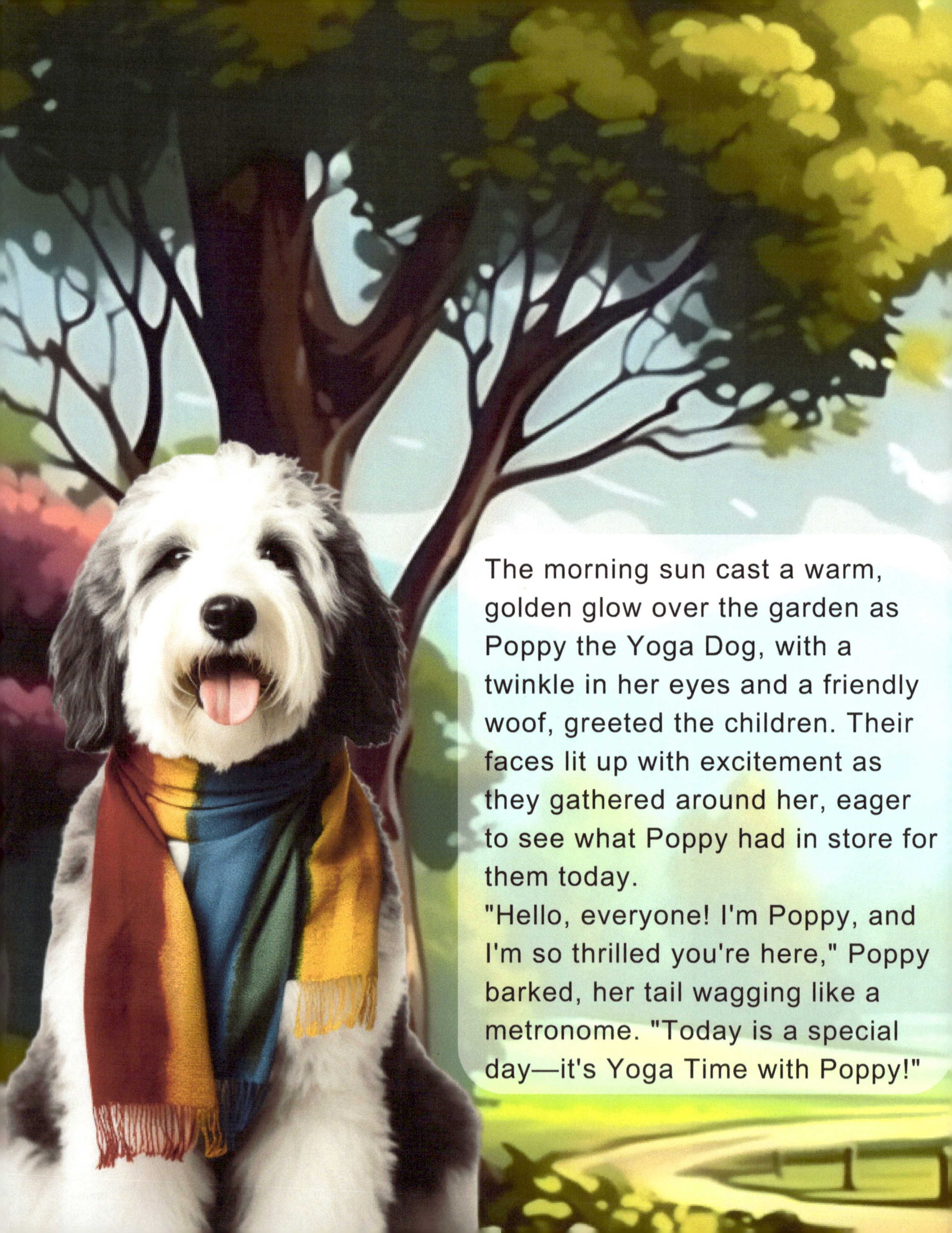
The morning sun cast a warm, golden glow over the garden as Poppy the Yoga Dog, with a twinkle in her eyes and a friendly woof, greeted the children. Their faces lit up with excitement as they gathered around her, eager to see what Poppy had in store for them today.
"Hello, everyone! I'm Poppy, and I'm so thrilled you're here," Poppy barked, her tail wagging like a metronome. "Today is a special day—it's Yoga Time with Poppy!"

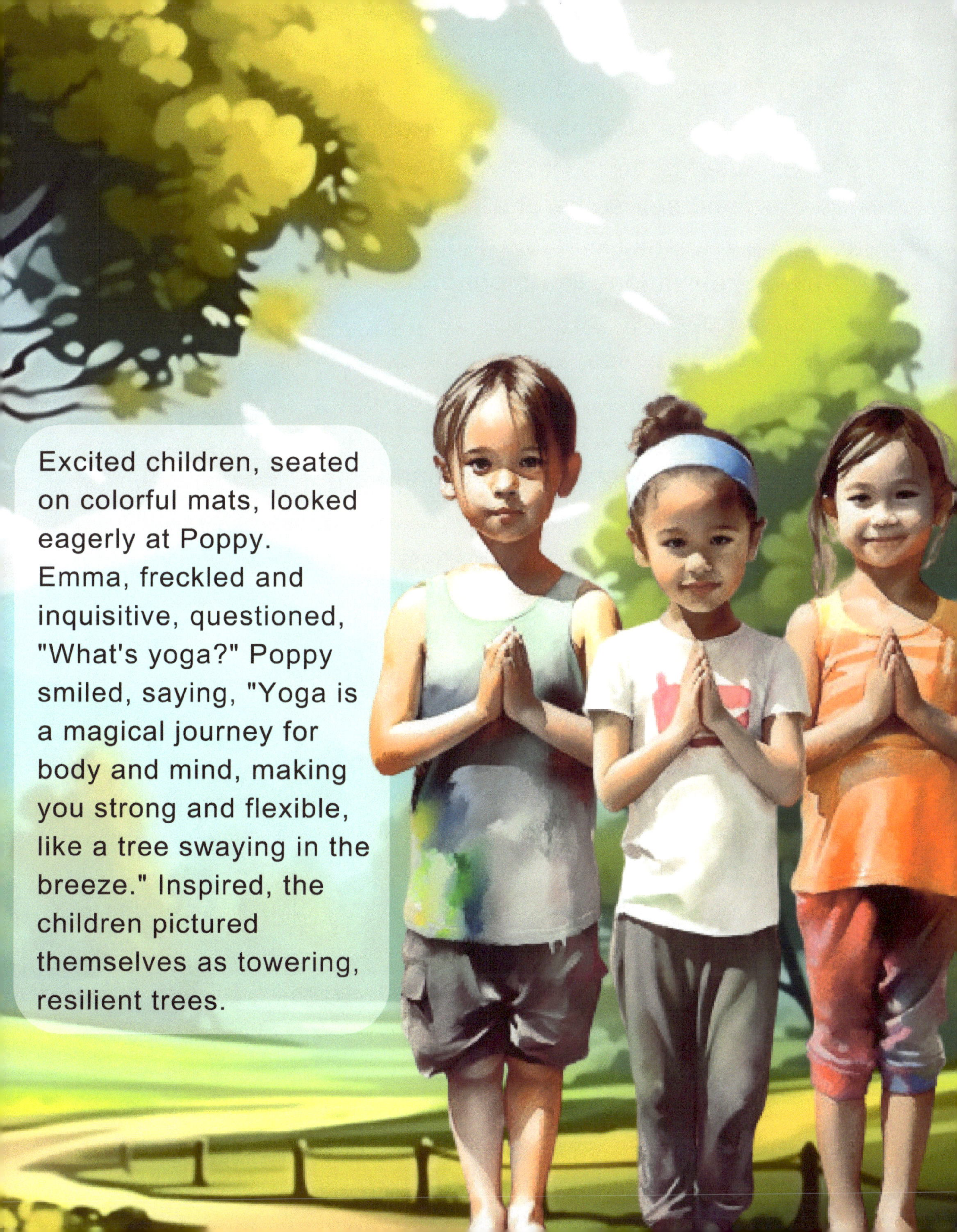

Excited children, seated on colorful mats, looked eagerly at Poppy. Emma, freckled and inquisitive, questioned, "What's yoga?" Poppy smiled, saying, "Yoga is a magical journey for body and mind, making you strong and flexible, like a tree swaying in the breeze." Inspired, the children pictured themselves as towering, resilient trees.

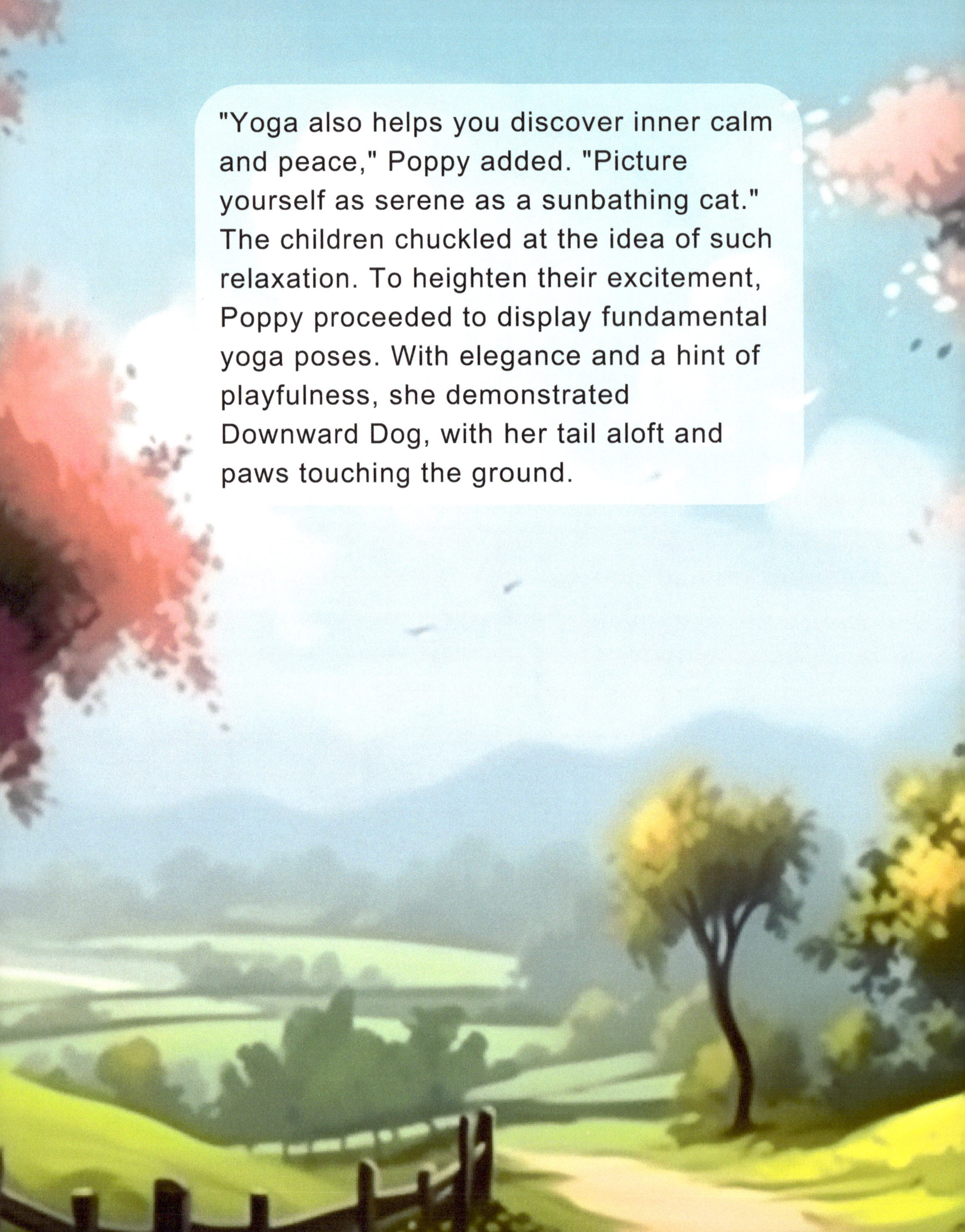

"Yoga also helps you discover inner calm and peace," Poppy added. "Picture yourself as serene as a sunbathing cat." The children chuckled at the idea of such relaxation. To heighten their excitement, Poppy proceeded to display fundamental yoga poses. With elegance and a hint of playfulness, she demonstrated Downward Dog, with her tail aloft and paws touching the ground.

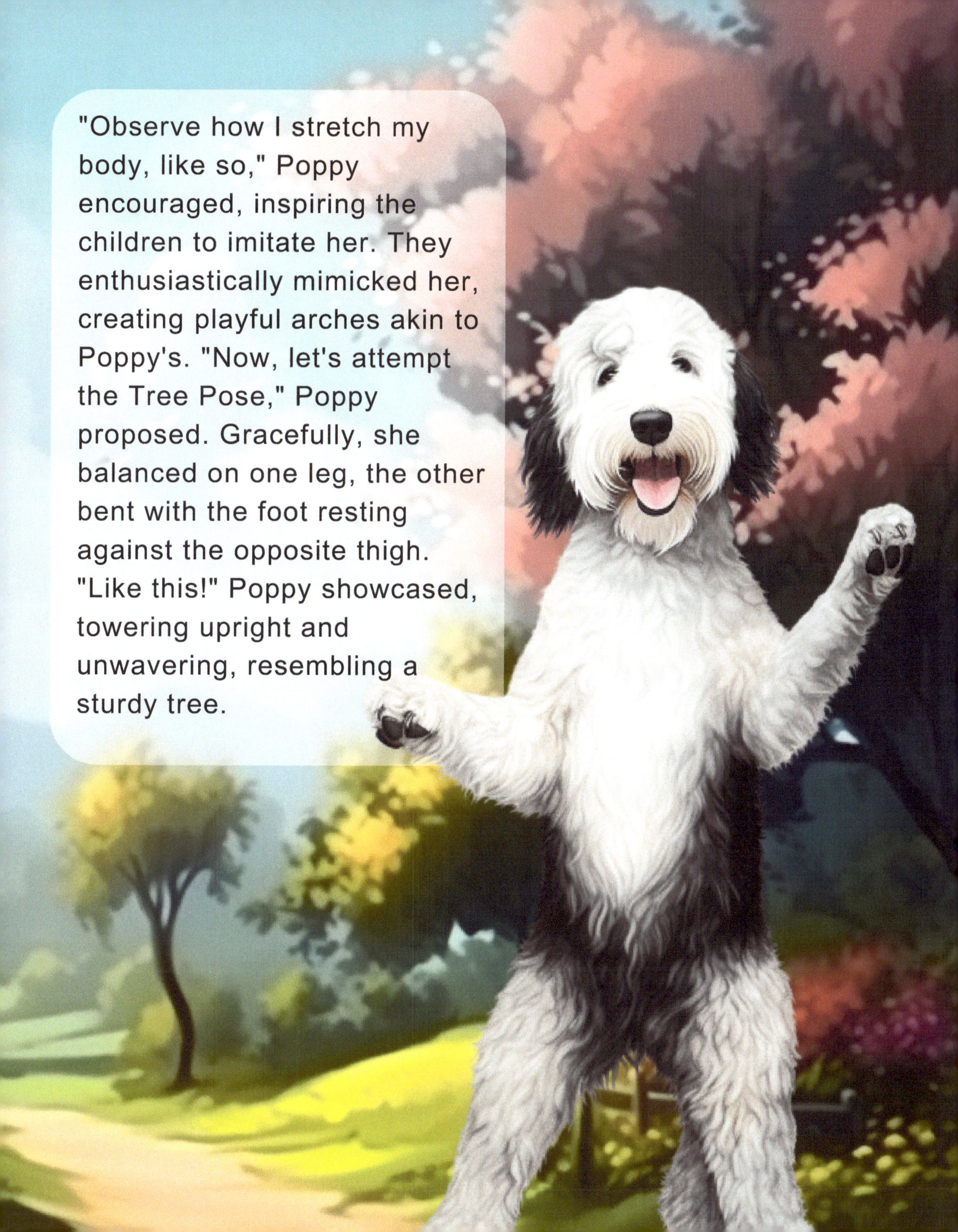

"Observe how I stretch my body, like so," Poppy encouraged, inspiring the children to imitate her. They enthusiastically mimicked her, creating playful arches akin to Poppy's. "Now, let's attempt the Tree Pose," Poppy proposed. Gracefully, she balanced on one leg, the other bent with the foot resting against the opposite thigh. "Like this!" Poppy showcased, towering upright and unwavering, resembling a sturdy tree.

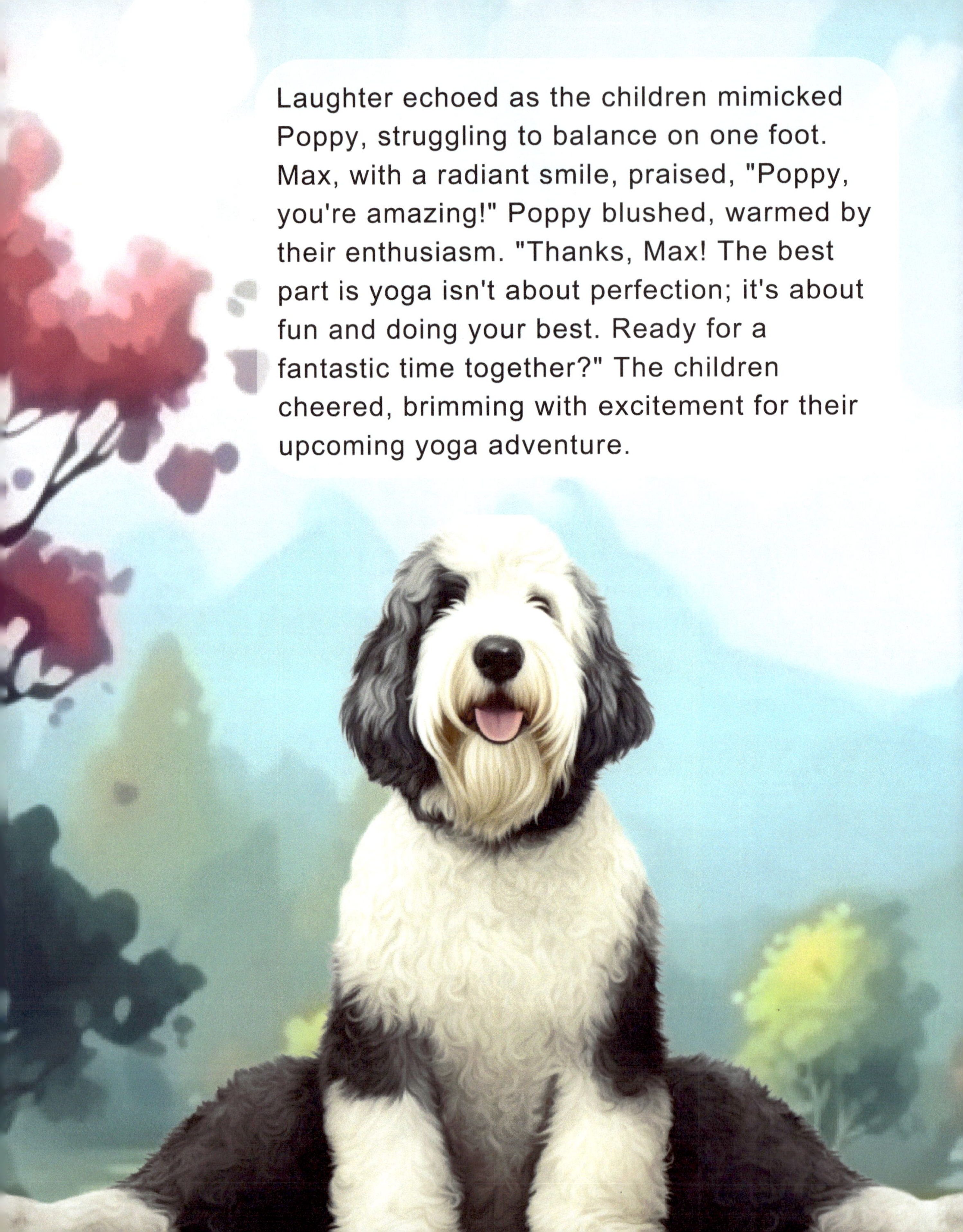

Laughter echoed as the children mimicked Poppy, struggling to balance on one foot. Max, with a radiant smile, praised, "Poppy, you're amazing!" Poppy blushed, warmed by their enthusiasm. "Thanks, Max! The best part is yoga isn't about perfection; it's about fun and doing your best. Ready for a fantastic time together?" The children cheered, brimming with excitement for their upcoming yoga adventure.

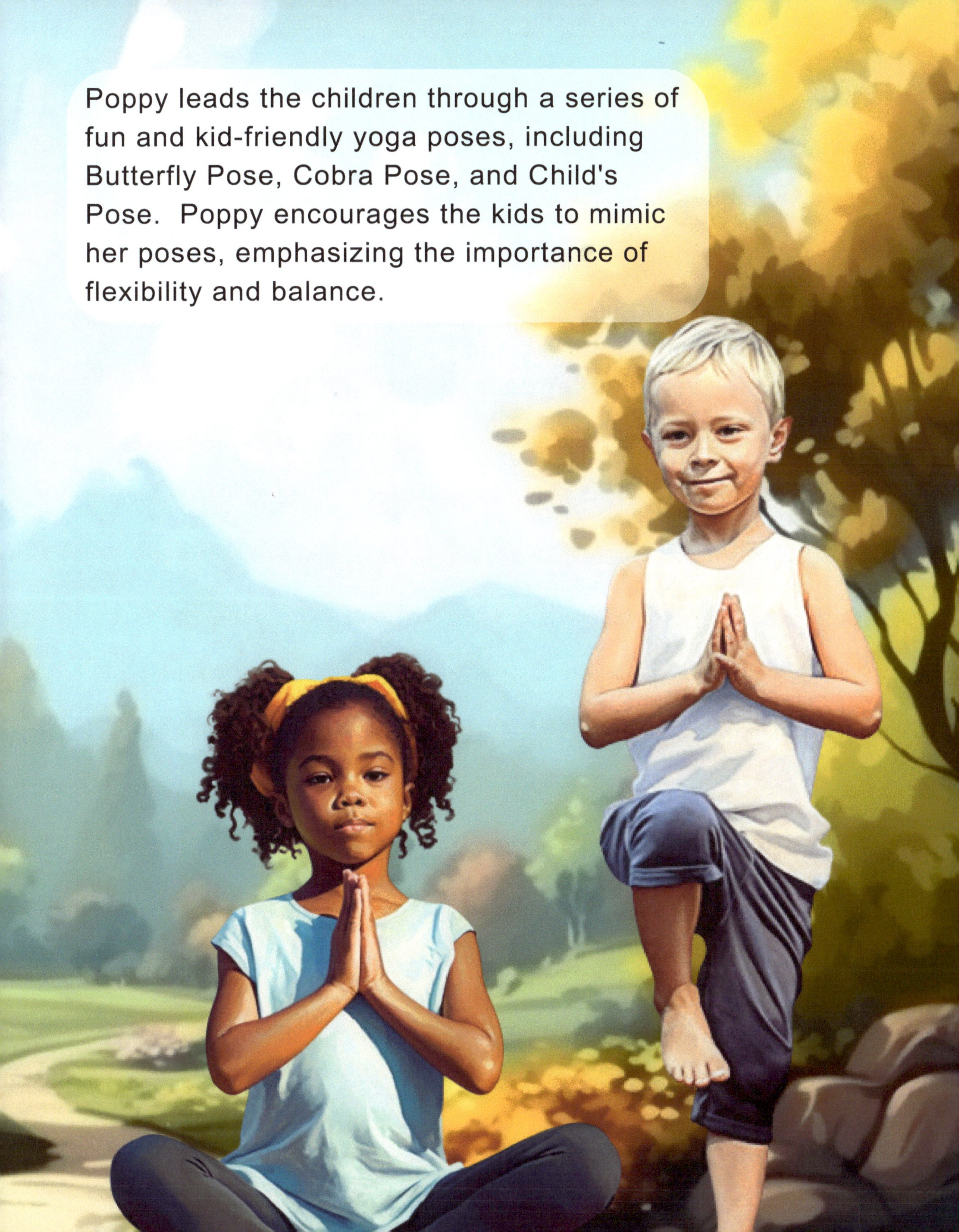
Poppy leads the children through a series of fun and kid-friendly yoga poses, including Butterfly Pose, Cobra Pose, and Child's Pose. Poppy encourages the kids to mimic her poses, emphasizing the importance of flexibility and balance.

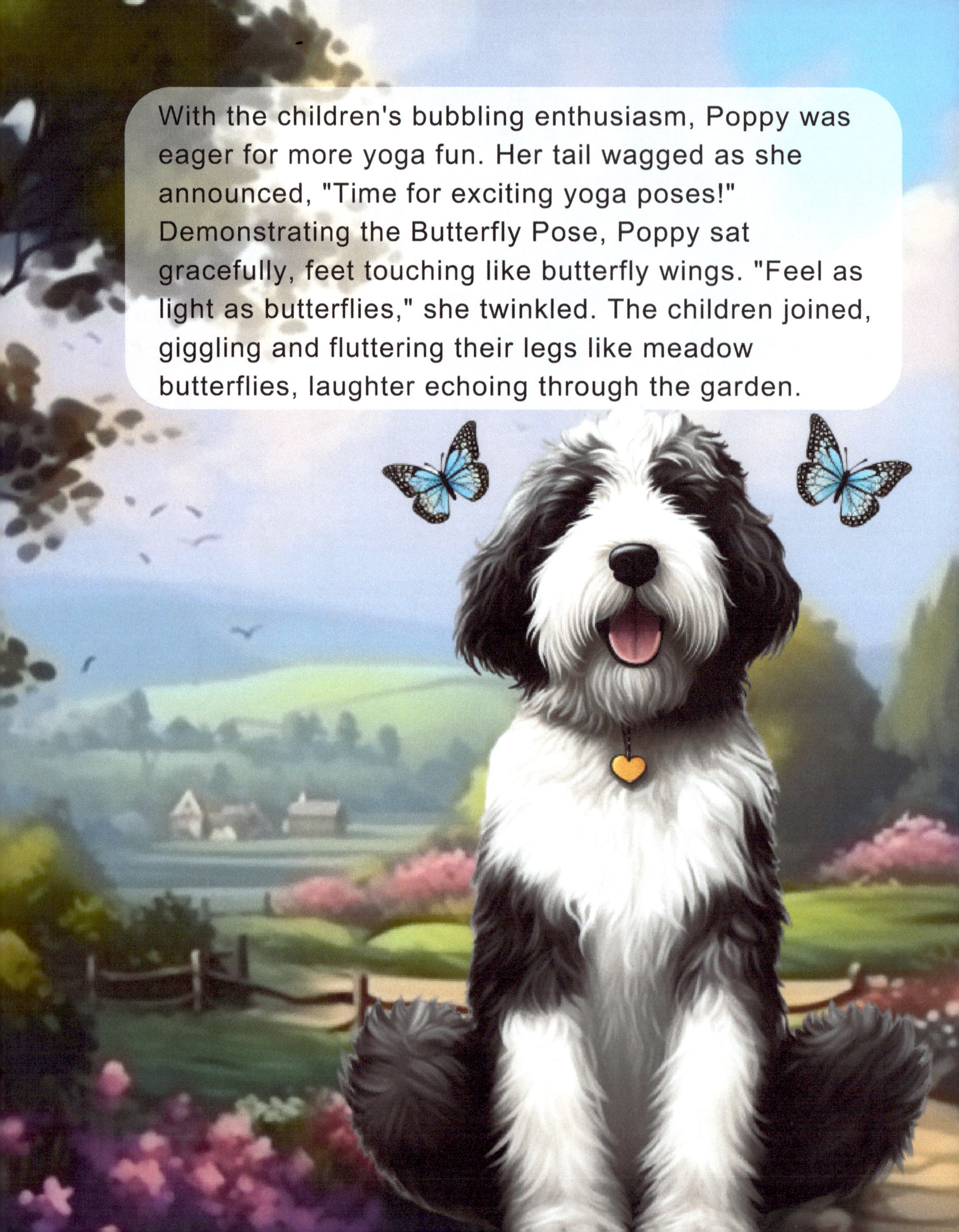

With the children's bubbling enthusiasm, Poppy was eager for more yoga fun. Her tail wagged as she announced, "Time for exciting yoga poses!" Demonstrating the Butterfly Pose, Poppy sat gracefully, feet touching like butterfly wings. "Feel as light as butterflies," she twinkled. The children joined, giggling and fluttering their legs like meadow butterflies, laughter echoing through the garden.

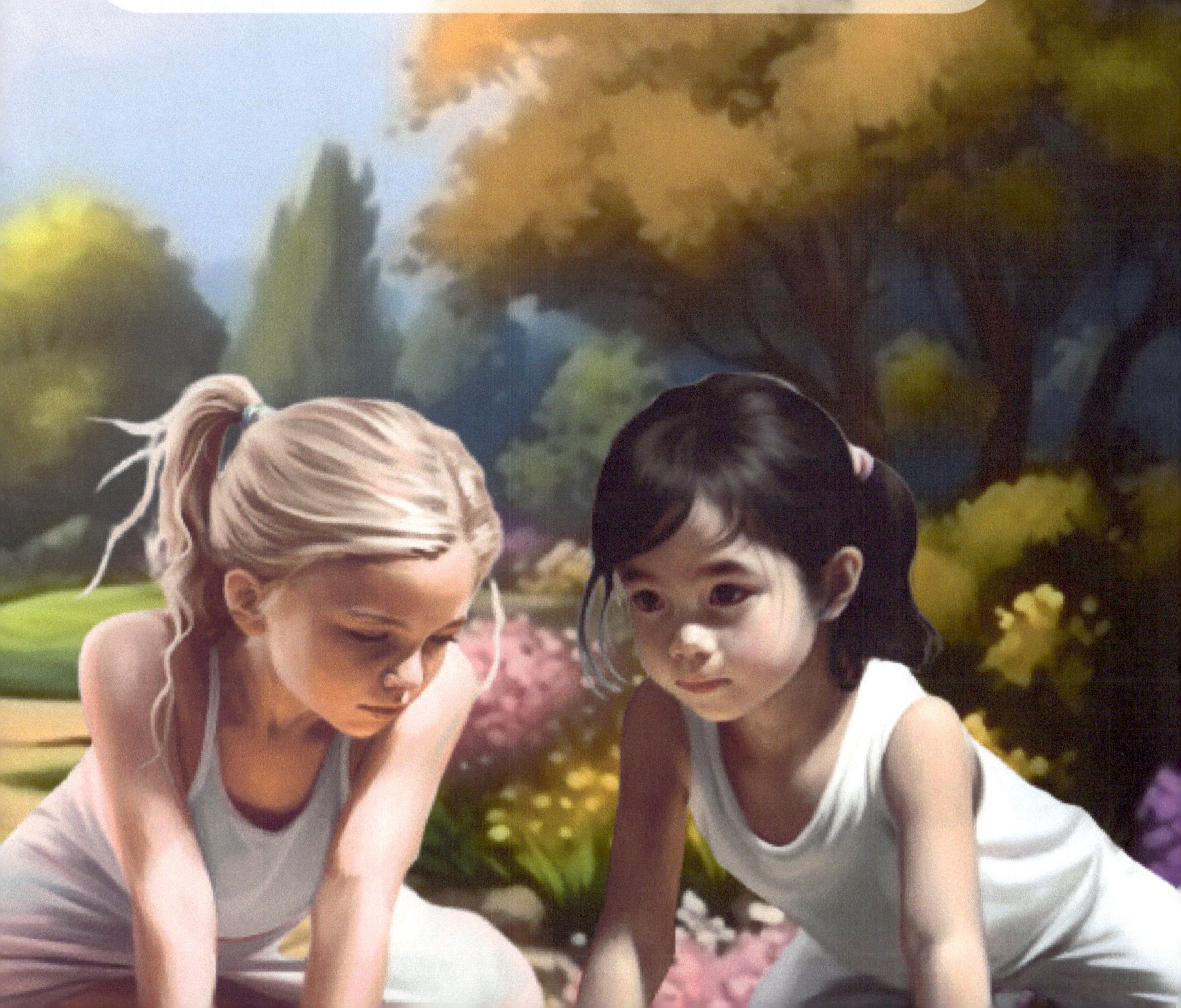

Cobra Pose: Poppy extended her body, low and elongated, lifting her head and chest like a cobra emerging from a basket. "The Cobra Pose," Poppy explained, "strengthens your spine and emboldens your heart. Give it a try!" The children imitated her, arching their backs and raising their heads high, envisioning themselves as fearless cobras, ready to explore the jungle's mysteries.

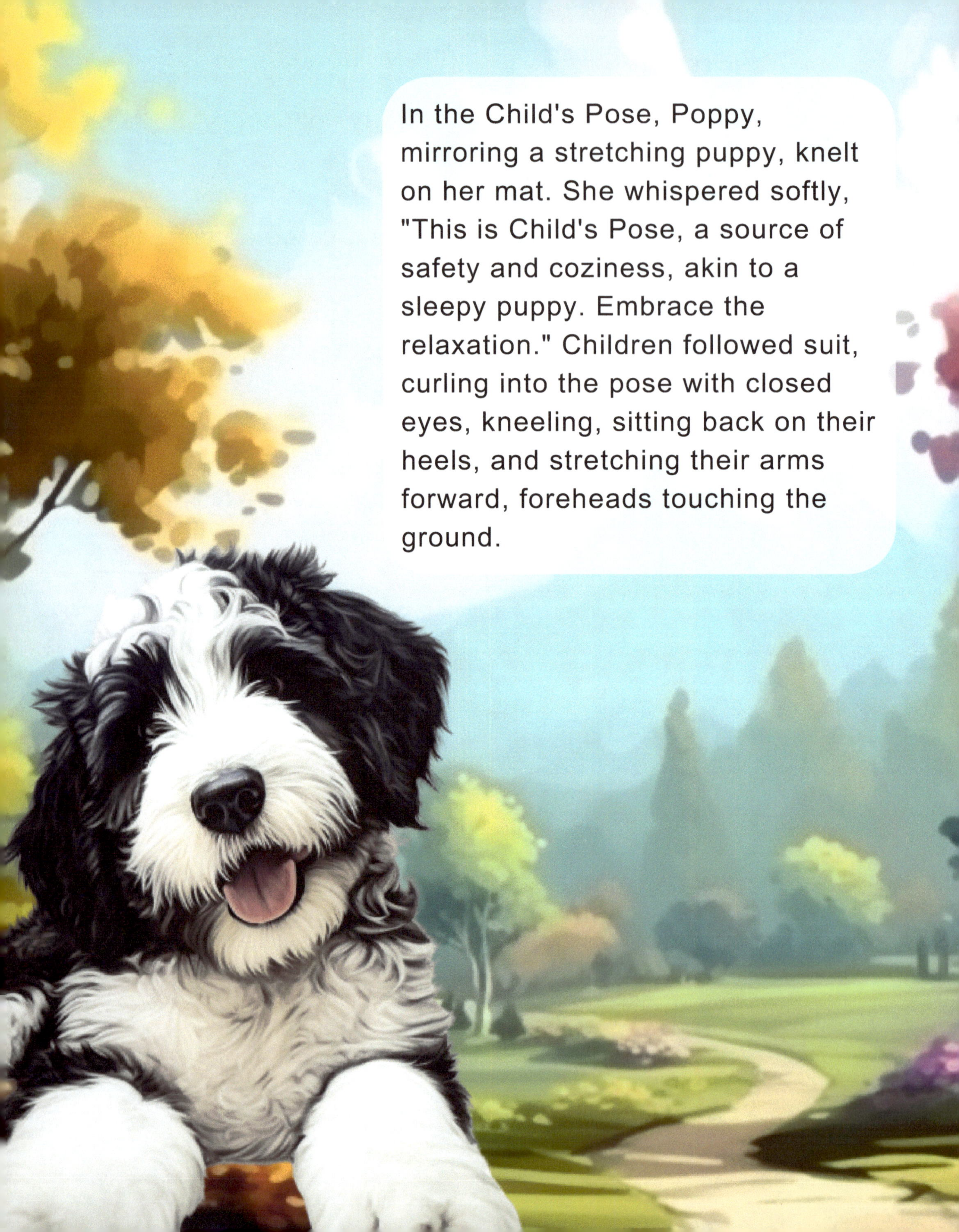

In the Child's Pose, Poppy, mirroring a stretching puppy, knelt on her mat. She whispered softly, "This is Child's Pose, a source of safety and coziness, akin to a sleepy puppy. Embrace the relaxation." Children followed suit, curling into the pose with closed eyes, kneeling, sitting back on their heels, and stretching their arms forward, foreheads touching the ground.

Tree Pose: Stand on one leg and place the sole of the other foot on the inner thigh of the standing leg.

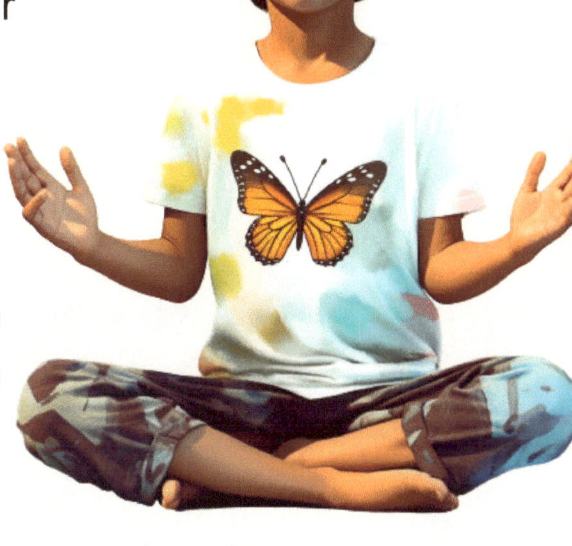

Butterfly Pose: Sit with the soles of the feet together, knees bent outward, and gently flap the legs like butterfly wings.

Downward Dog: Begin on hands and knees, then lift the hips up and back, forming an inverted V shape.

"Great job, everyone!" Poppy cheered. "Yoga means strength, flexibility, and fun. No right or wrong way—just be yourself and enjoy!"

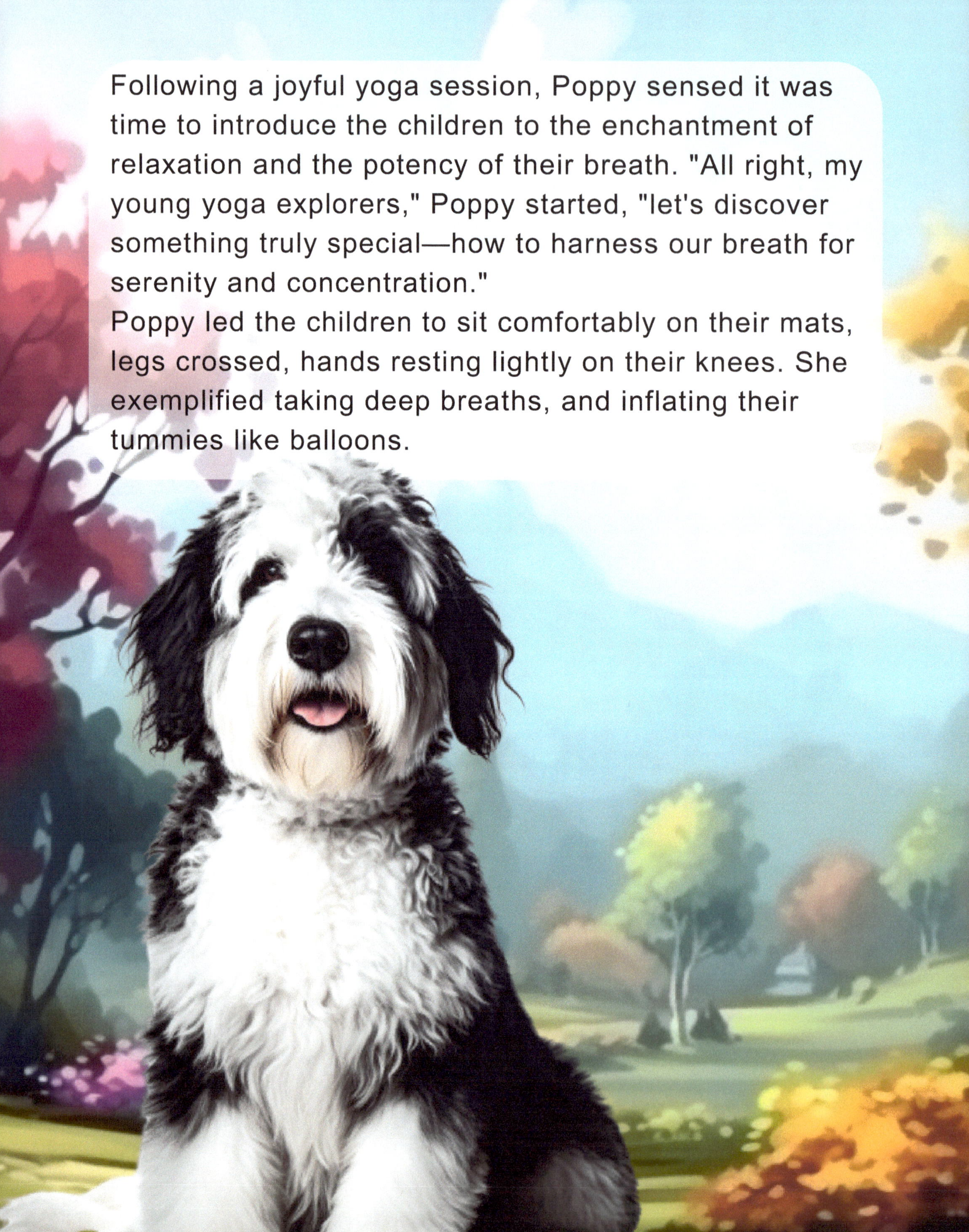
Following a joyful yoga session, Poppy sensed it was time to introduce the children to the enchantment of relaxation and the potency of their breath. "All right, my young yoga explorers," Poppy started, "let's discover something truly special—how to harness our breath for serenity and concentration."
Poppy led the children to sit comfortably on their mats, legs crossed, hands resting lightly on their knees. She exemplified taking deep breaths, and inflating their tummies like balloons.

"Let's practice deep belly breathing," Poppy's smile radiated serenity. "Imagine your tummy as a balloon. Inhale and your balloon expands; exhale, and it contracts."
The children mimicked, inhaling through their noses, their tummies ballooning, then exhaling gently. Their rhythmic breaths harmonized, creating a tranquil garden melody.
"Great job," Poppy praised. "This breath brings calm and readiness; use it for inner peace when needed."

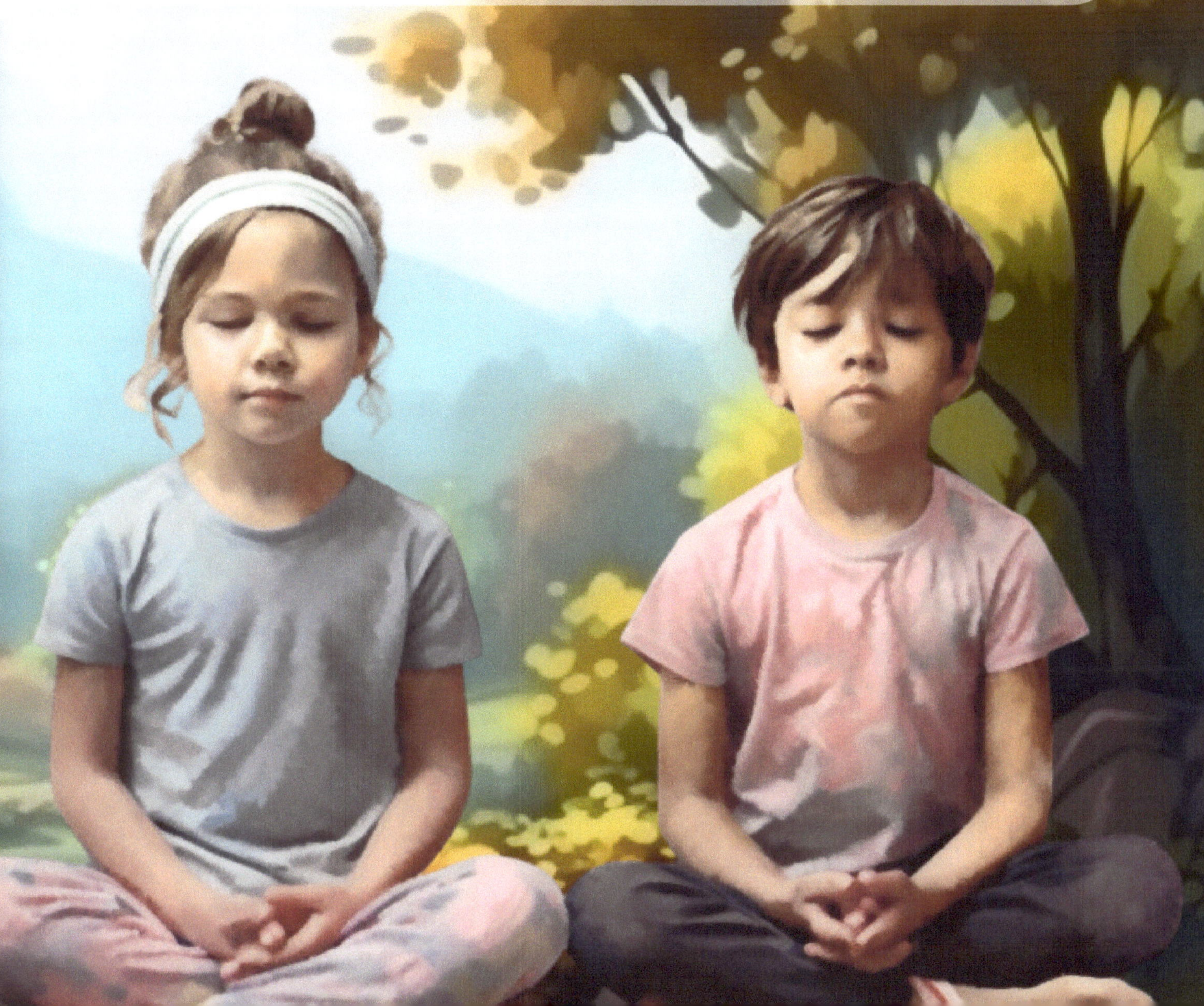

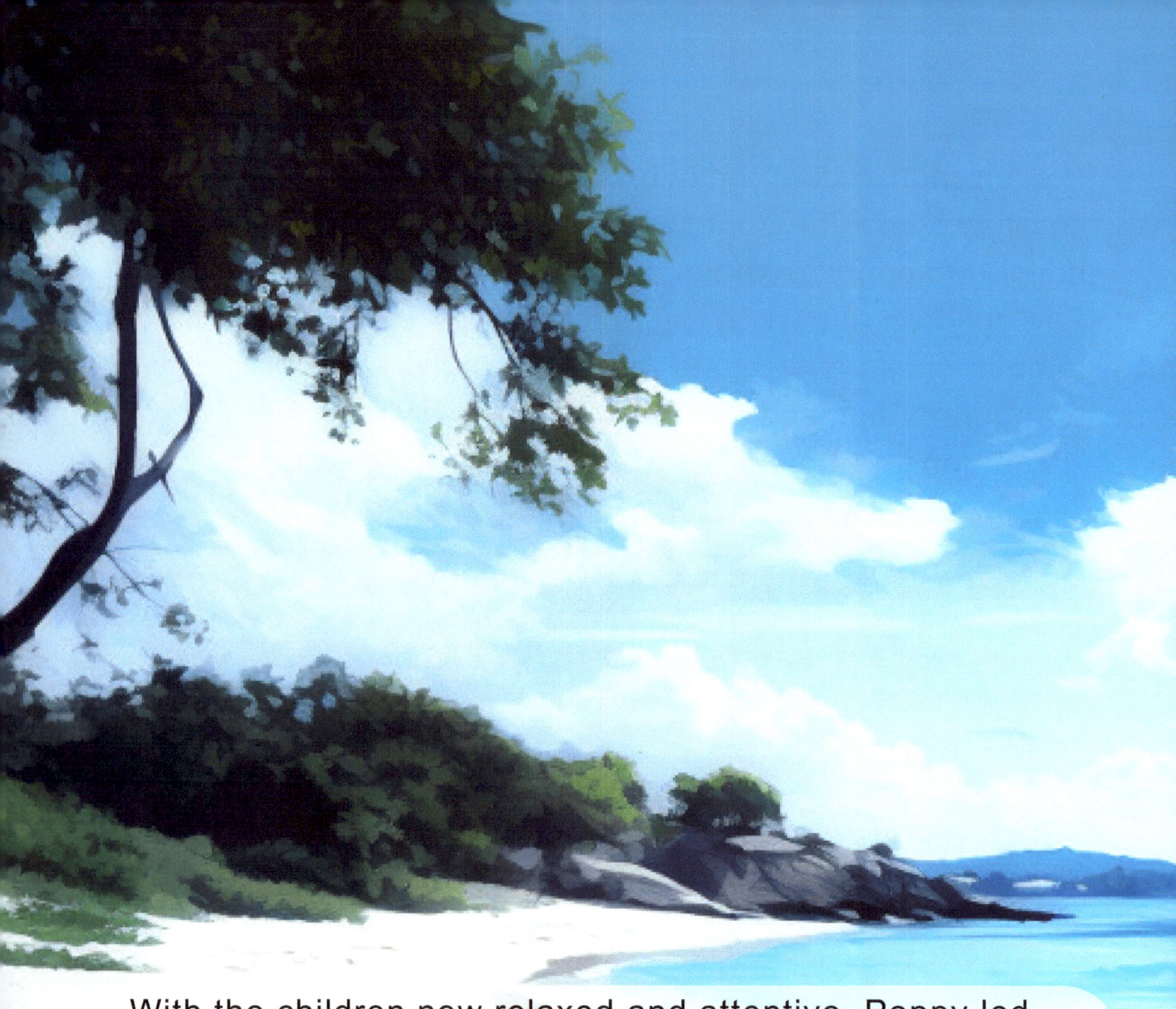

With the children now relaxed and attentive, Poppy led them on a magical journey using their imagination. "Close your eyes," she whispered, "and envision the most serene place you can think of—a tranquil beach, a cozy forest, or drifting among the stars."

As the children closed their eyes, Poppy's gentle voice persisted, "Imagine every detail—colors, sounds, scents. Inhale deeply, feel the tranquility infusing you. As you exhale, release worries and tension."

In a quiet garden, all you could hear were the soft sounds of leaves rustling and Poppy's gentle voice. The kids were sitting comfortably, feeling very happy. Poppy whispered, "Whenever life gets too busy, close your eyes and find your special peaceful place inside. It's always there for you."

After a little more time, Poppy said, "Now, slowly open your eyes. Great job, little yoga explorers! Just remember, your breath and your imagination are like magic keys that can make you feel happy and calm."

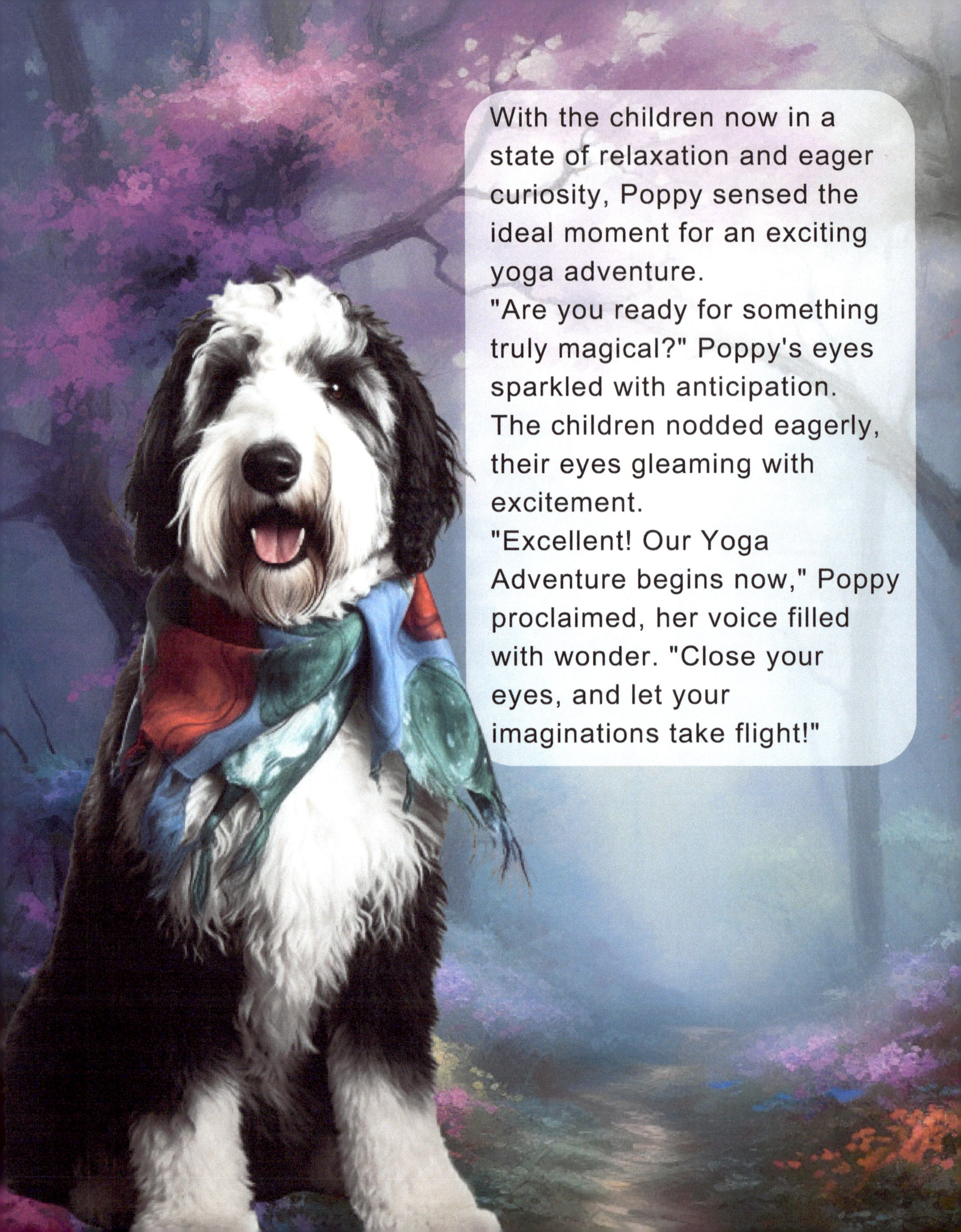

With the children now in a state of relaxation and eager curiosity, Poppy sensed the ideal moment for an exciting yoga adventure.
"Are you ready for something truly magical?" Poppy's eyes sparkled with anticipation.
The children nodded eagerly, their eyes gleaming with excitement.
"Excellent! Our Yoga Adventure begins now," Poppy proclaimed, her voice filled with wonder. "Close your eyes, and let your imaginations take flight!"

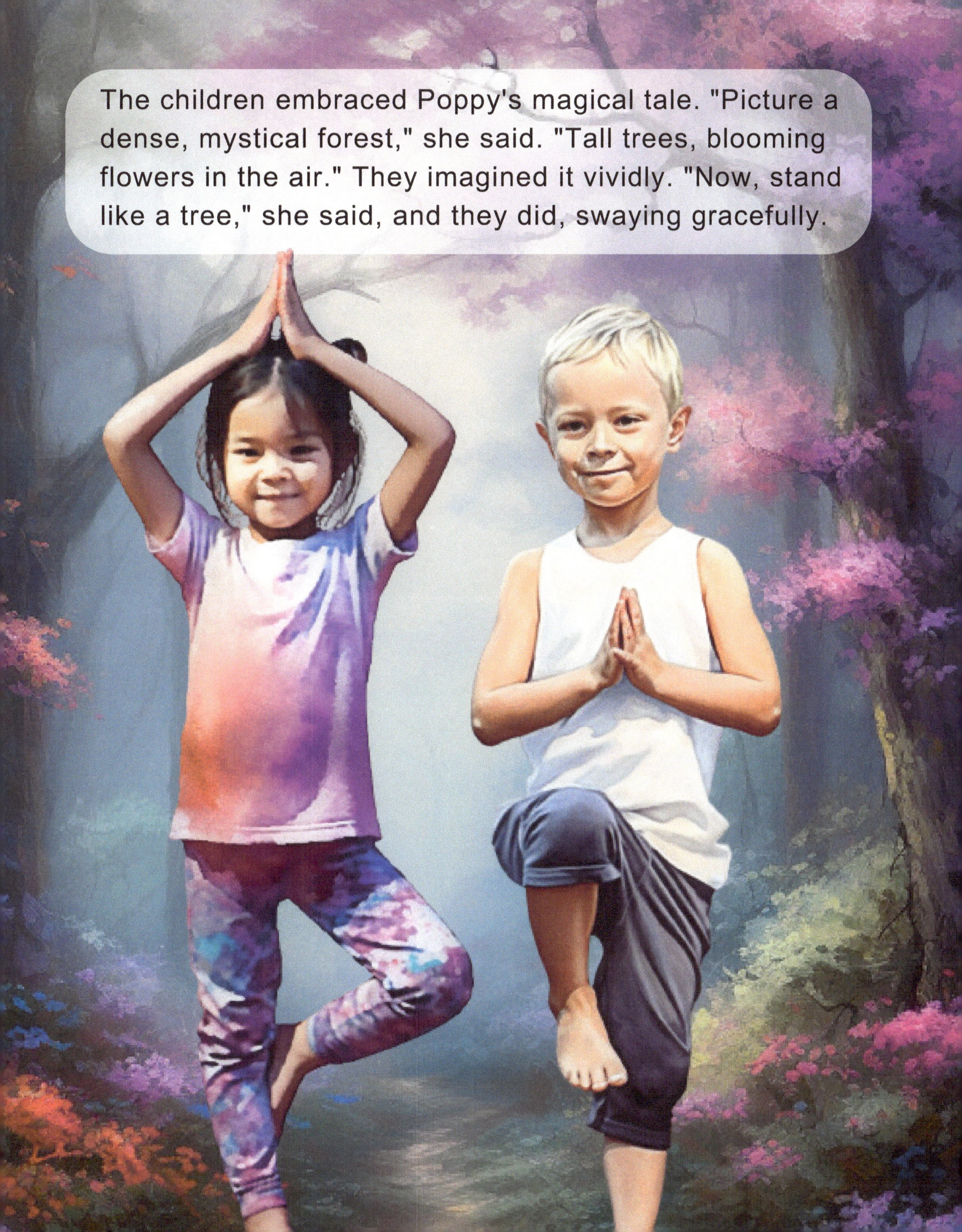
The children embraced Poppy's magical tale. "Picture a dense, mystical forest," she said. "Tall trees, blooming flowers in the air." They imagined it vividly. "Now, stand like a tree," she said, and they did, swaying gracefully.

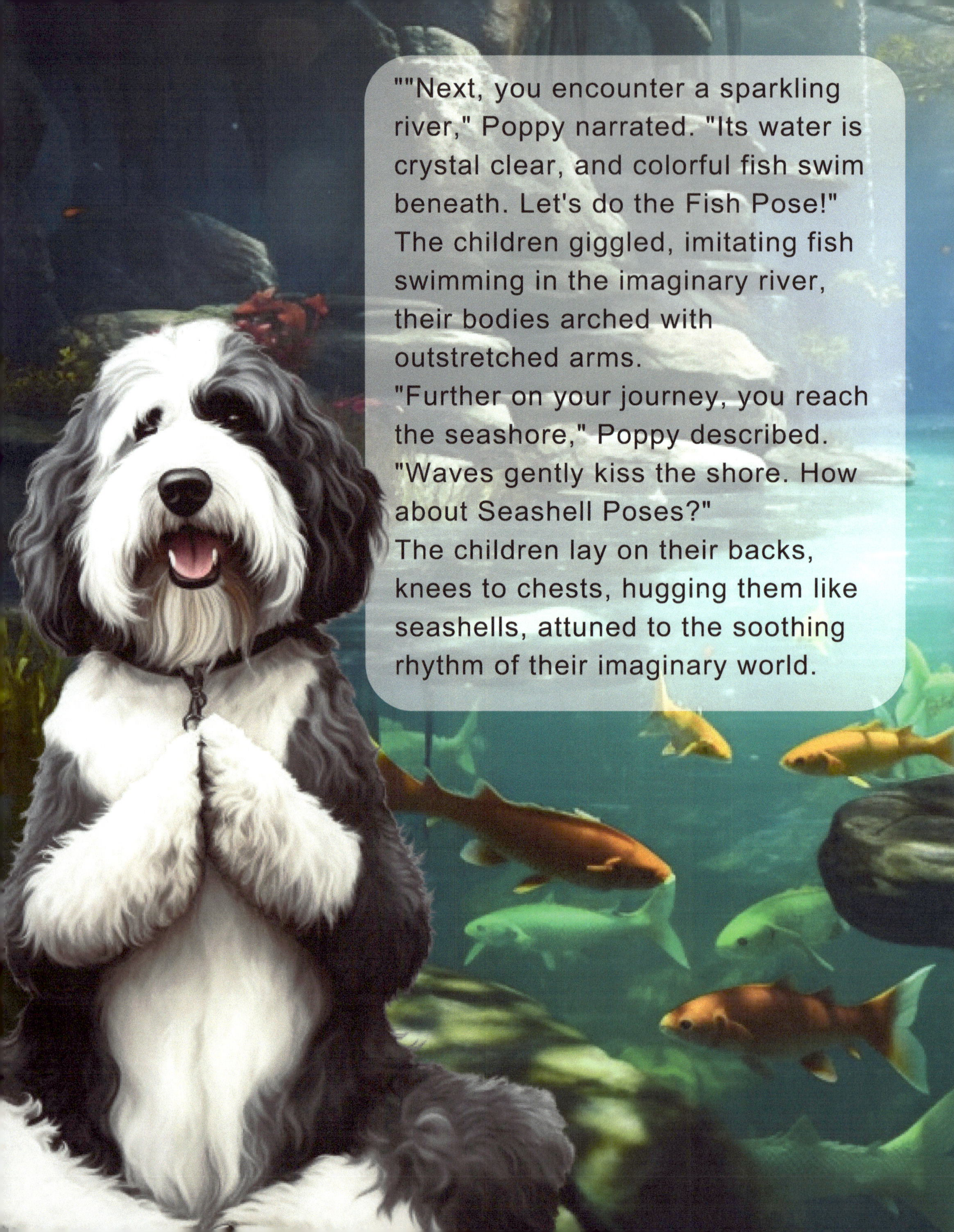
""Next, you encounter a sparkling river," Poppy narrated. "Its water is crystal clear, and colorful fish swim beneath. Let's do the Fish Pose!"
The children giggled, imitating fish swimming in the imaginary river, their bodies arched with outstretched arms.
"Further on your journey, you reach the seashore," Poppy described. "Waves gently kiss the shore. How about Seashell Poses?"
The children lay on their backs, knees to chests, hugging them like seashells, attuned to the soothing rhythm of their imaginary world.

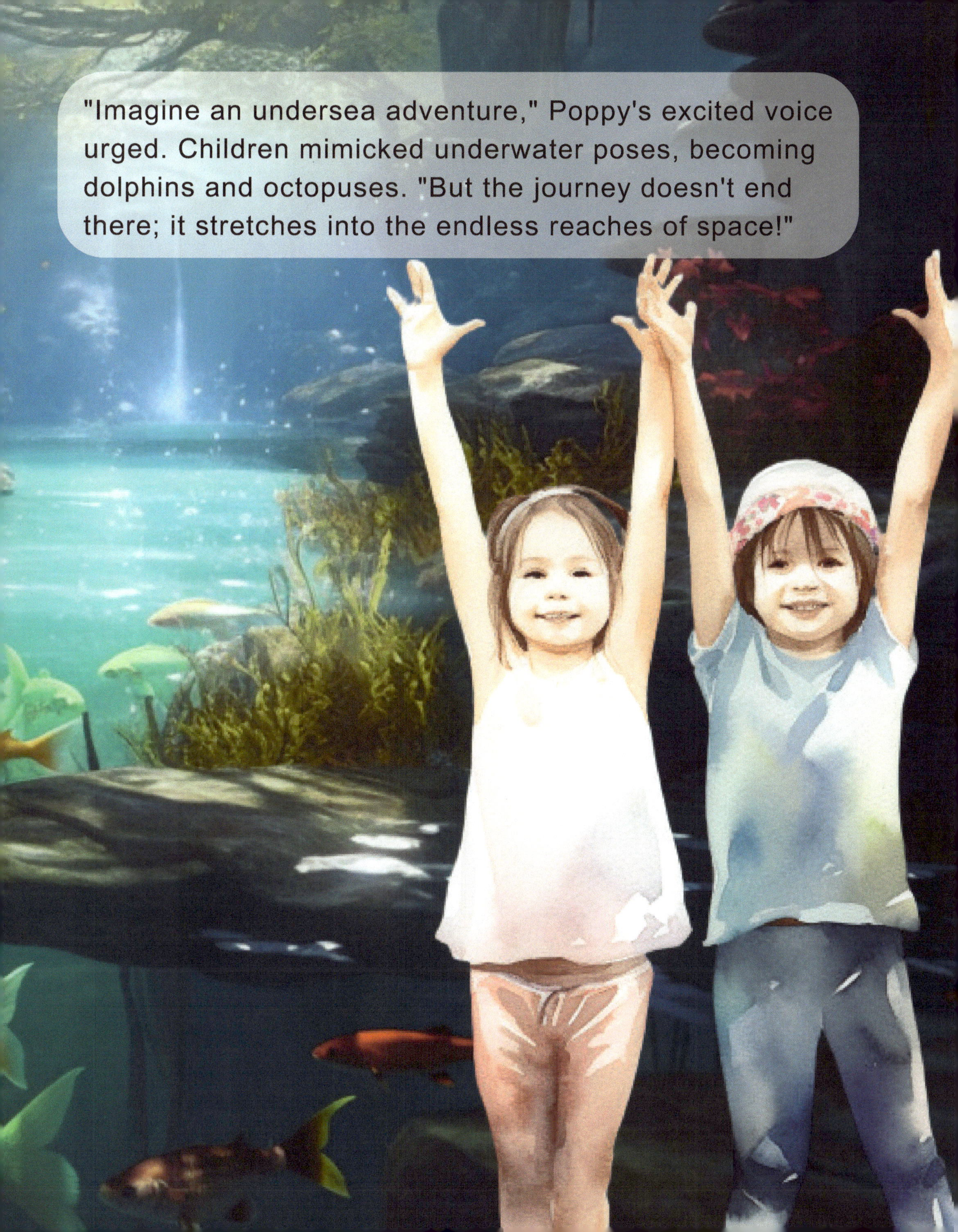

"Imagine an undersea adventure," Poppy's excited voice urged. Children mimicked underwater poses, becoming dolphins and octopuses. "But the journey doesn't end there; it stretches into the endless reaches of space!"

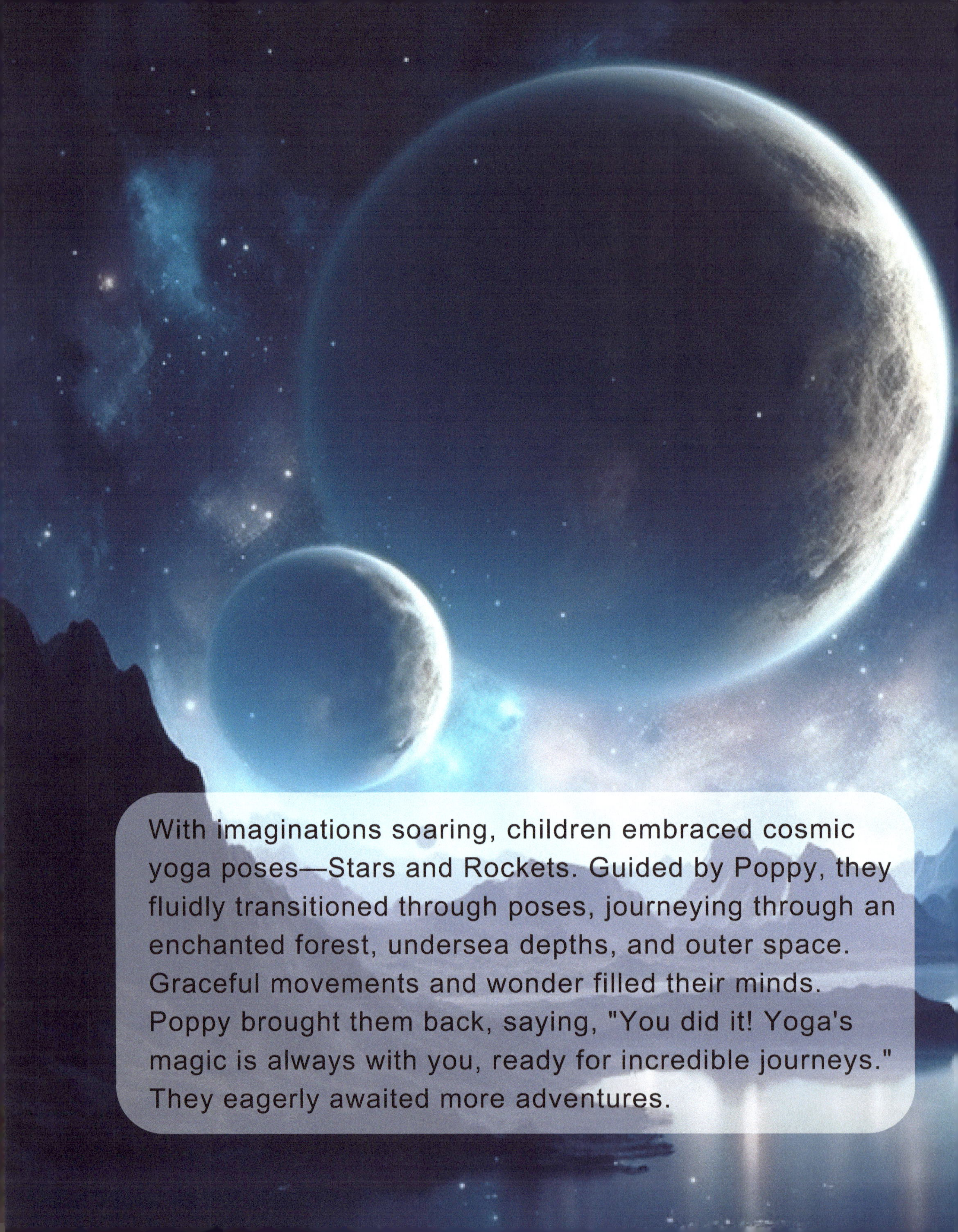

With imaginations soaring, children embraced cosmic yoga poses—Stars and Rockets. Guided by Poppy, they fluidly transitioned through poses, journeying through an enchanted forest, undersea depths, and outer space. Graceful movements and wonder filled their minds. Poppy brought them back, saying, "You did it! Yoga's magic is always with you, ready for incredible journeys." They eagerly awaited more adventures.

Following their thrilling yoga odyssey through the enchanted forest, undersea depths, and outer space, Poppy assembled the children in a circle on their mats. They radiated excitement, their hearts enchanted by the journey.

"Now, after our incredible Yoga Adventure," Poppy started, "let's discuss some of yoga's fantastic benefits."

With warmth in her eyes, she regarded each child.

"Yoga strengthens and flexes our bodies, akin to the forest's resilient trees. It aids us in moving with grace and ease."

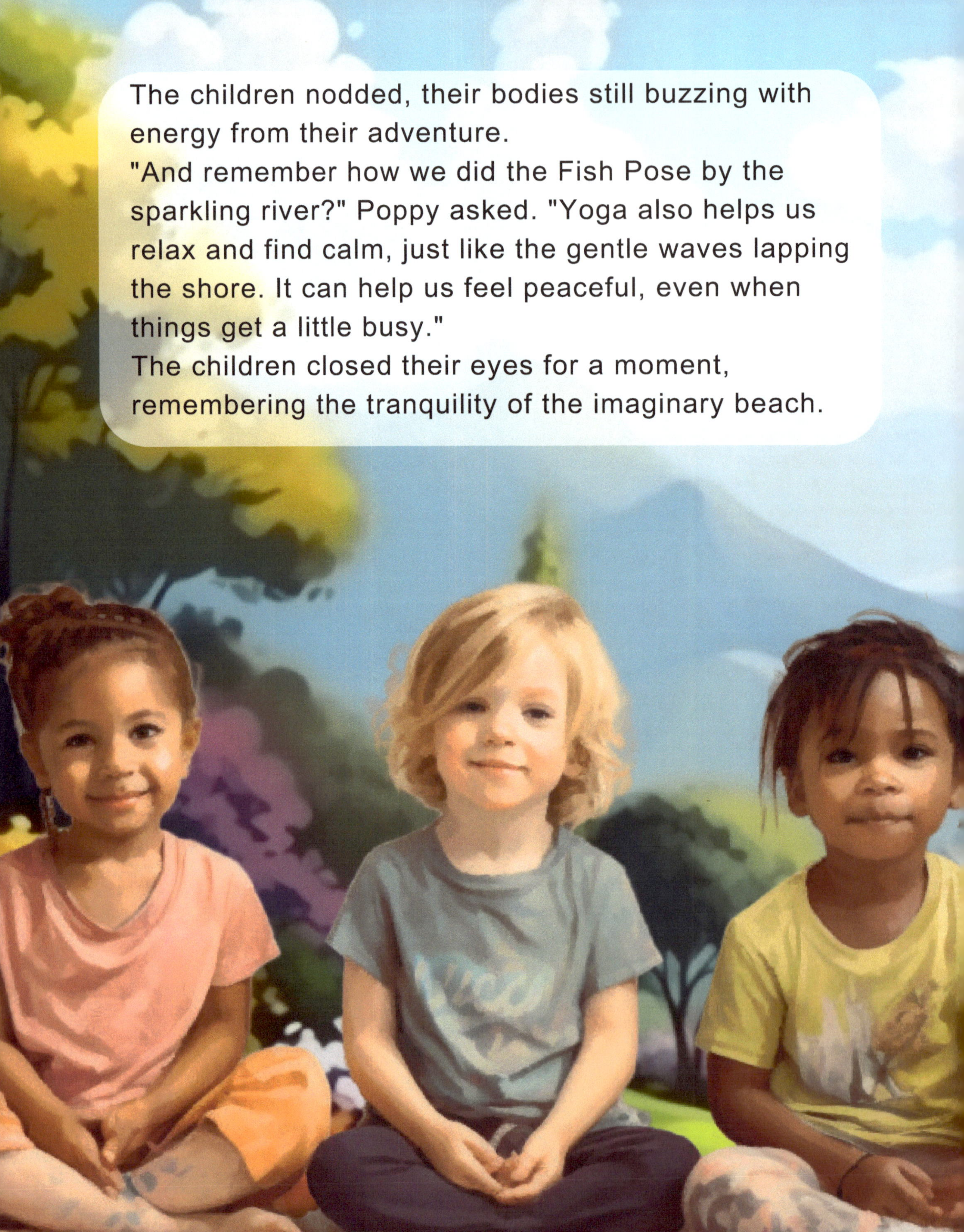

The children nodded, their bodies still buzzing with energy from their adventure.

"And remember how we did the Fish Pose by the sparkling river?" Poppy asked. "Yoga also helps us relax and find calm, just like the gentle waves lapping the shore. It can help us feel peaceful, even when things get a little busy."

The children closed their eyes for a moment, remembering the tranquility of the imaginary beach.

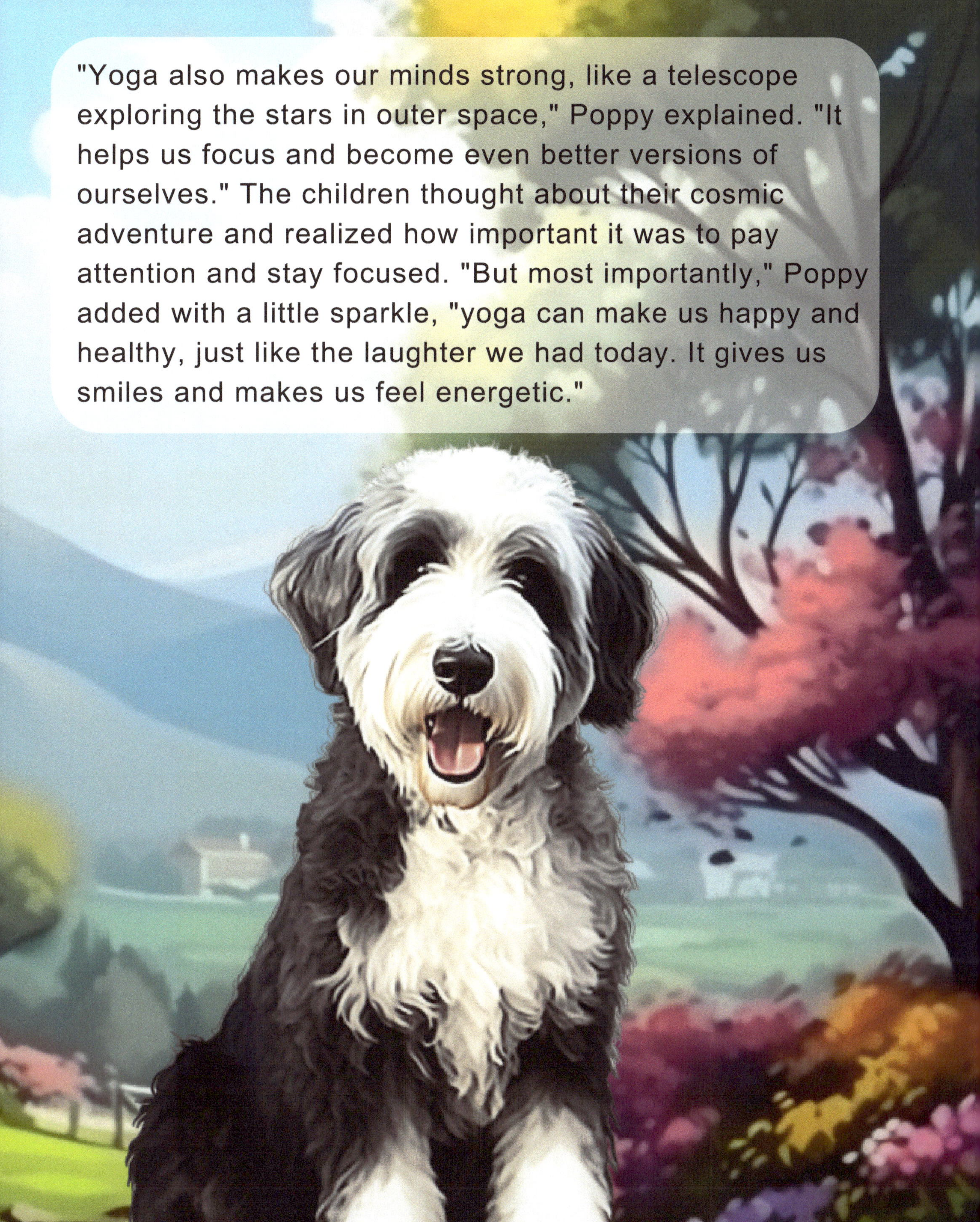
"Yoga also makes our minds strong, like a telescope exploring the stars in outer space," Poppy explained. "It helps us focus and become even better versions of ourselves." The children thought about their cosmic adventure and realized how important it was to pay attention and stay focused. "But most importantly," Poppy added with a little sparkle, "yoga can make us happy and healthy, just like the laughter we had today. It gives us smiles and makes us feel energetic."

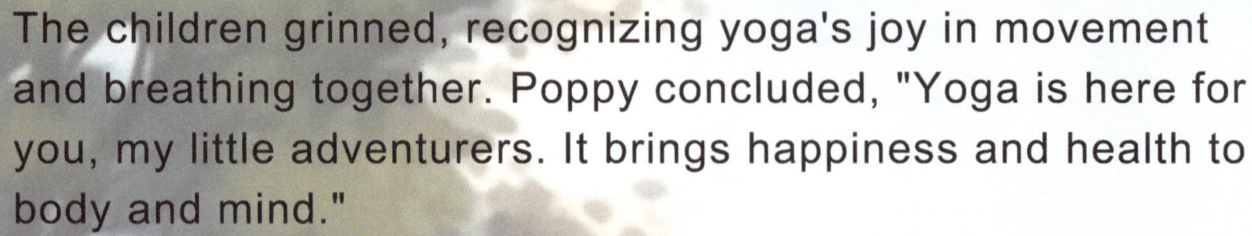

The children grinned, recognizing yoga's joy in movement and breathing together. Poppy concluded, "Yoga is here for you, my little adventurers. It brings happiness and health to body and mind."
Grateful hearts swelled for Poppy and yoga's newfound love. They felt a deep connection, aware of shared benefits. Sitting in their circle, they knew their adventures with Poppy were just beginning, with more exciting poses, stories, and benefits waiting to be discovered.

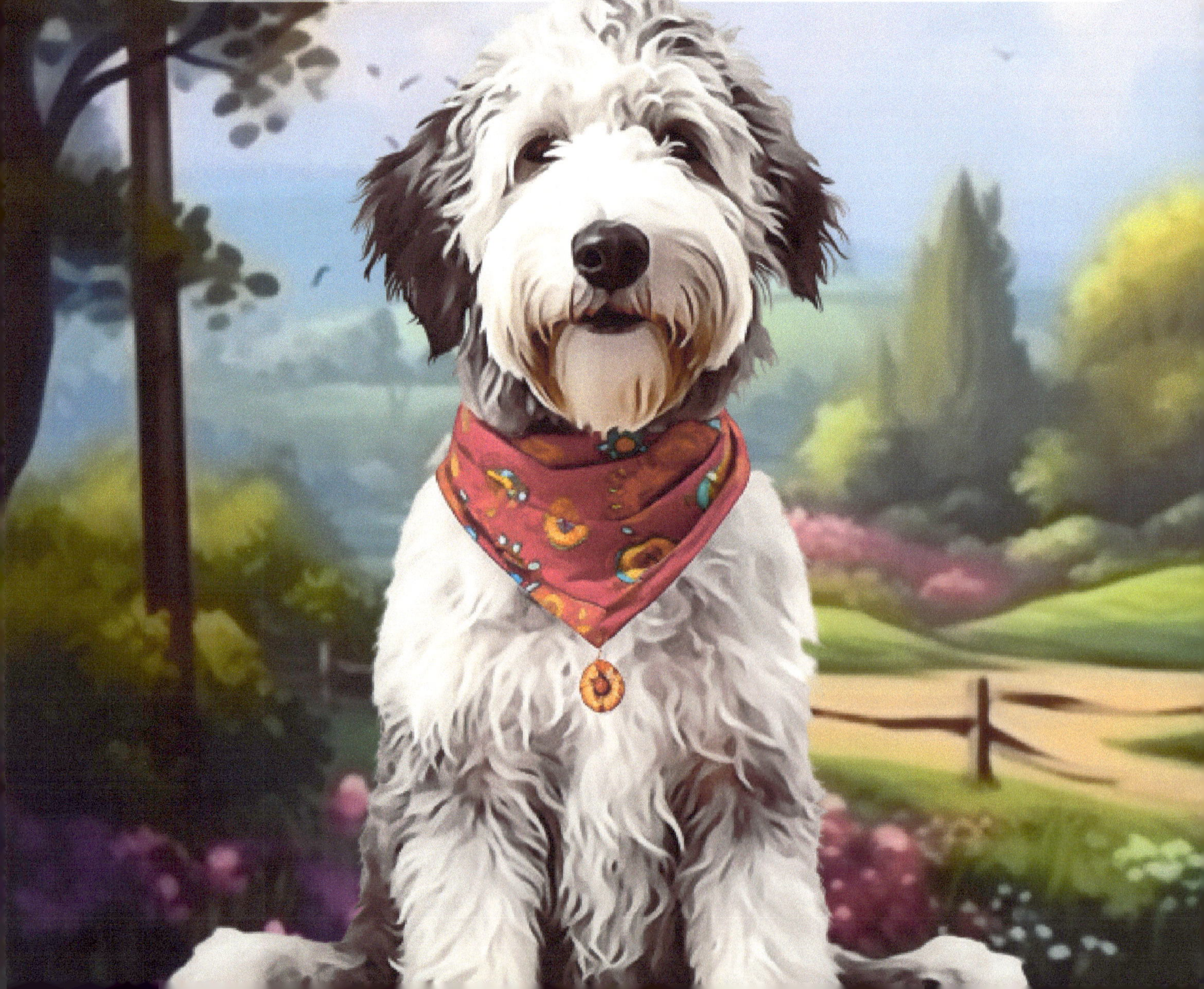

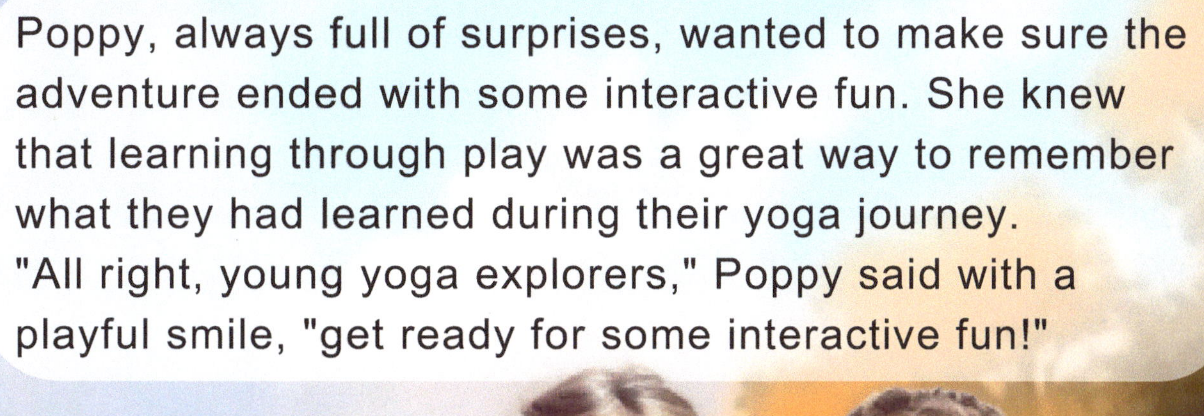

Poppy, always full of surprises, wanted to make sure the adventure ended with some interactive fun. She knew that learning through play was a great way to remember what they had learned during their yoga journey.
"All right, young yoga explorers," Poppy said with a playful smile, "get ready for some interactive fun!"

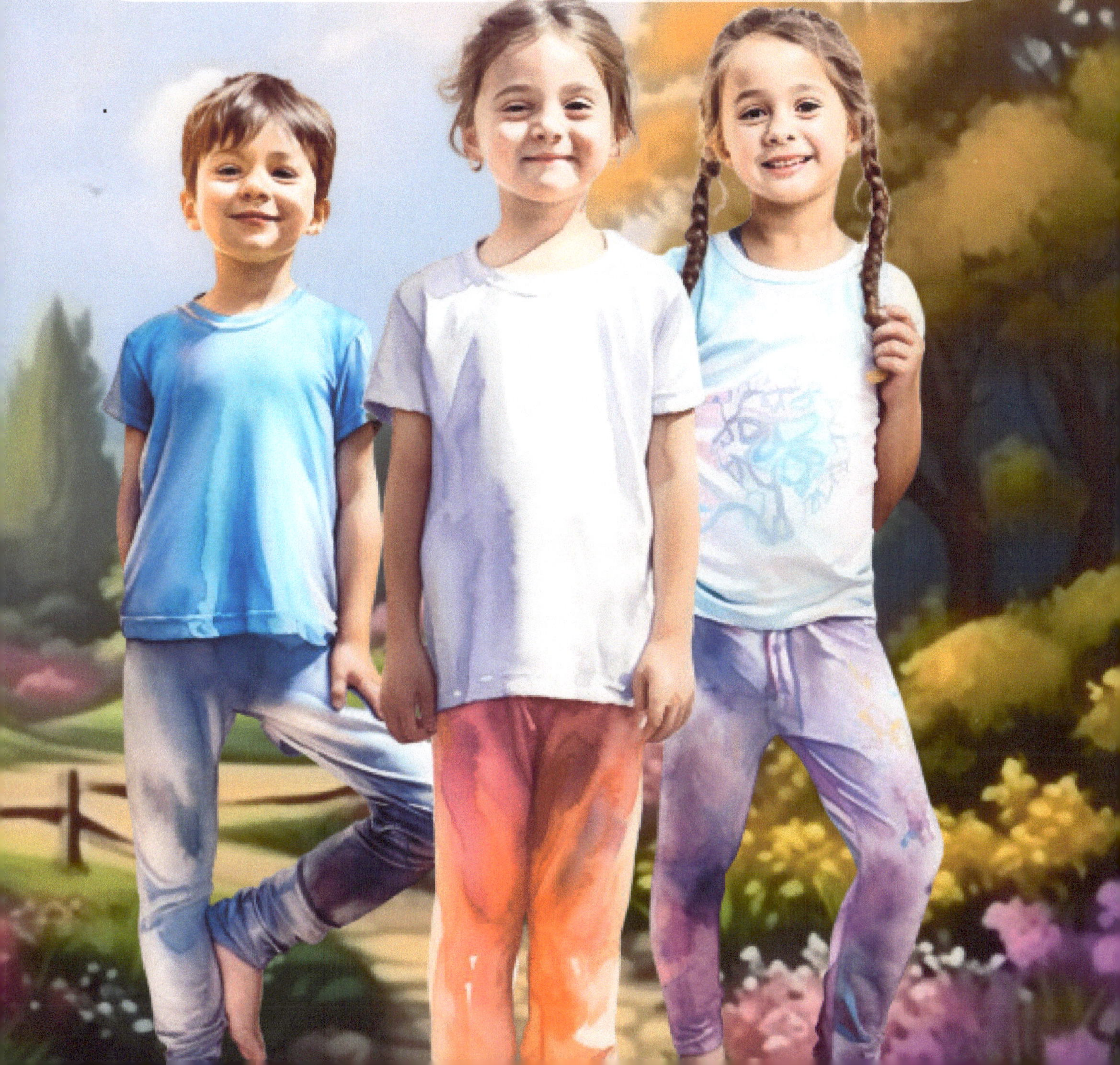

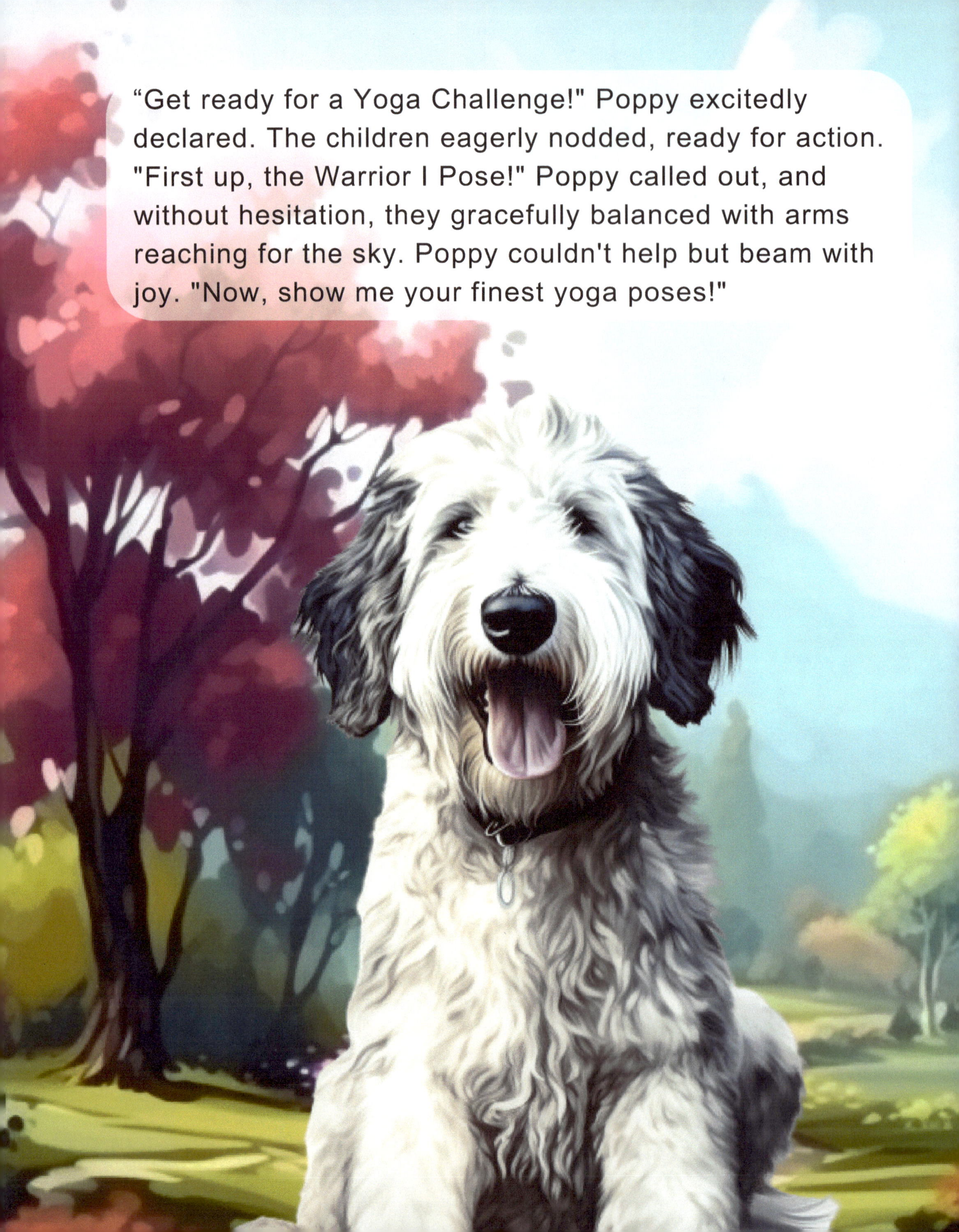

"Get ready for a Yoga Challenge!" Poppy excitedly declared. The children eagerly nodded, ready for action. "First up, the Warrior I Pose!" Poppy called out, and without hesitation, they gracefully balanced with arms reaching for the sky. Poppy couldn't help but beam with joy. "Now, show me your finest yoga poses!"

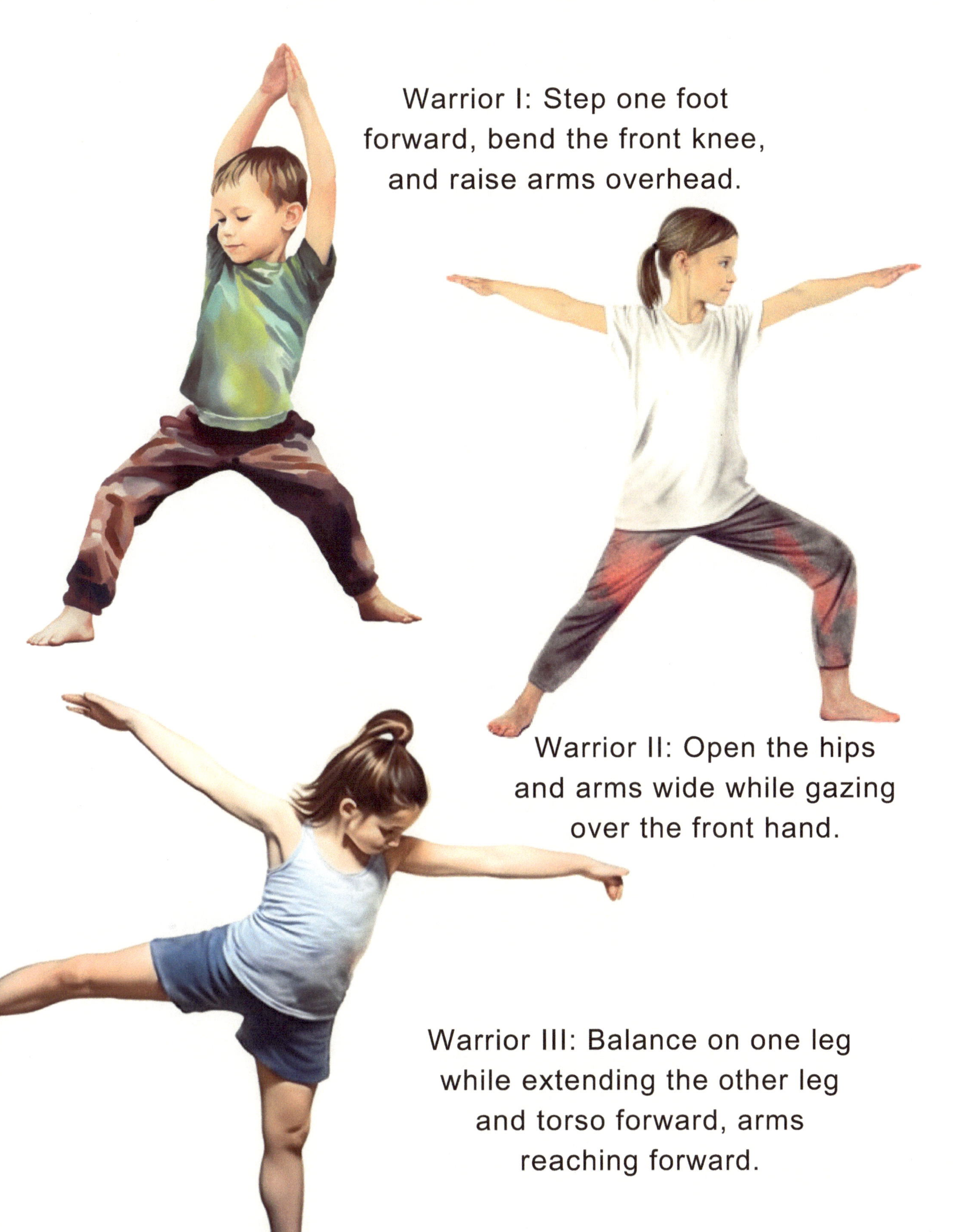

Warrior I: Step one foot forward, bend the front knee, and raise arms overhead.
Warrior II: Open the hips and arms wide while gazing over the front hand.
Warrior III: Balance on one leg while extending the other leg and torso forward, arms reaching forward.

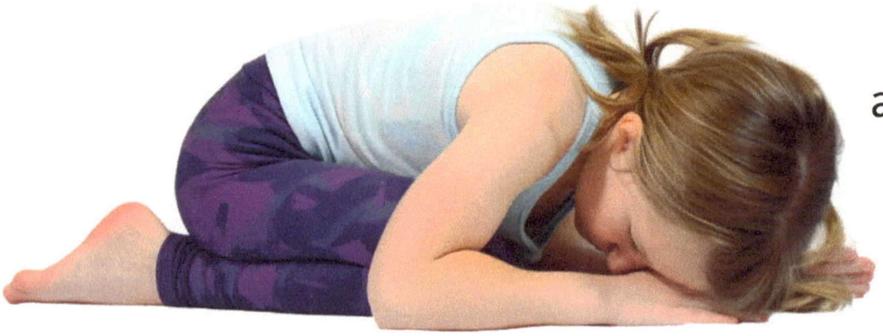

Child's Pose: Kneel on the floor, sit back on their heels, and stretch their arms forward with their forehead touching the ground.

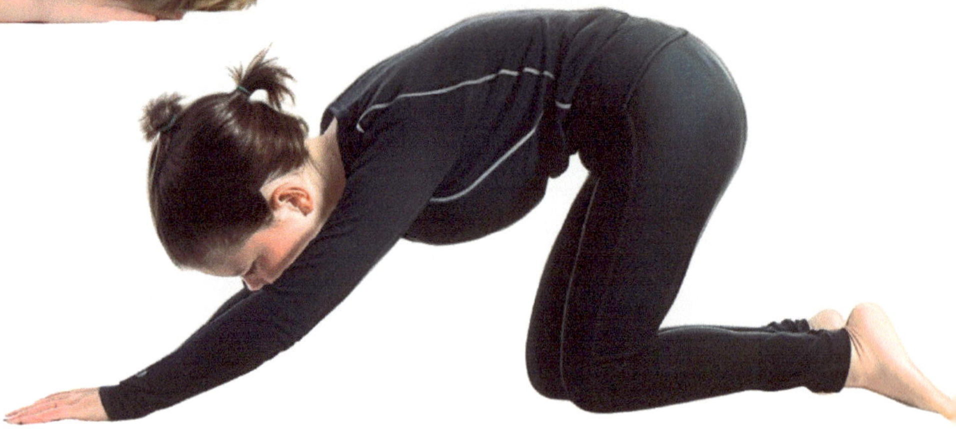

Cat-Cow Pose: Great for flexibility and spinal health. On hands and knees, arch the back upwards (cat pose) and then arch it downwards (cow pose).

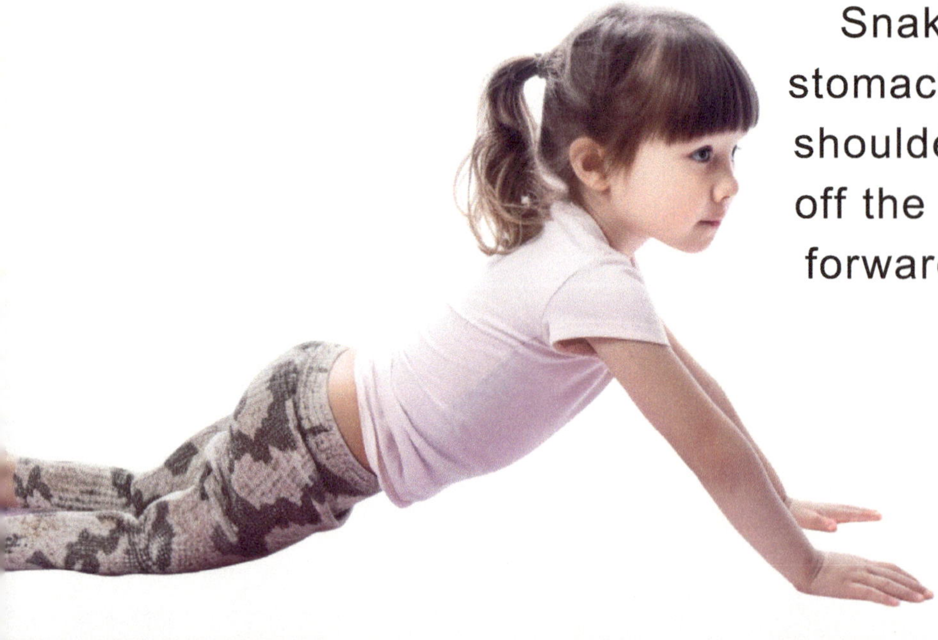

Snake Pose: Lie on the stomach, place hands under shoulders, and lift the chest off the ground while looking forward. Imagine slithering like a snake.

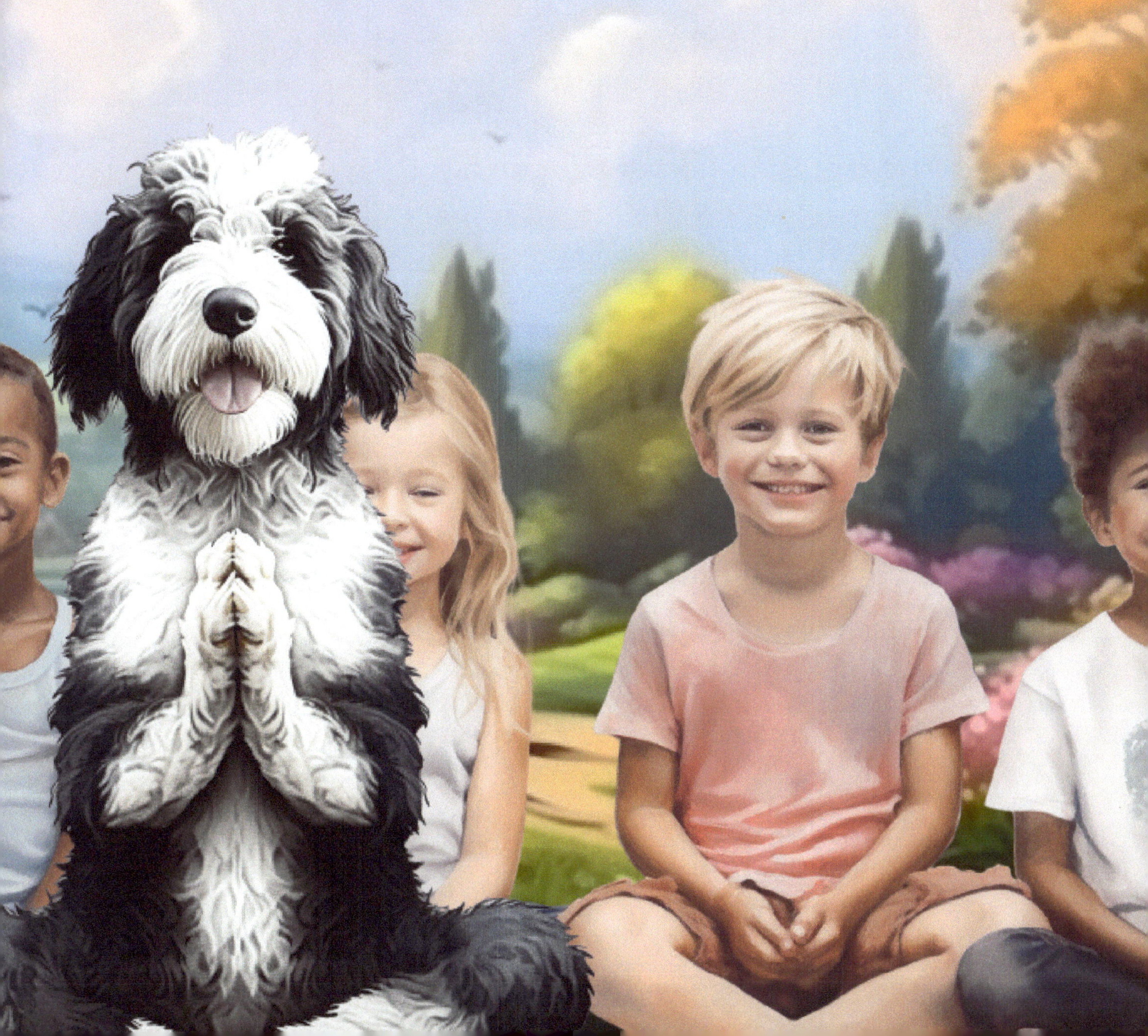
As the sun set, Poppy gathered the children in a final mat-bound circle. Hearts filled with memories from their yoga adventures. Poppy smiled, saying, "Goodbye for now, but remember, yoga is a lifelong treasure." Gratitude filled the air. "Thank you," whispered a child, and they left, hearts full, eager for more yoga. Namaste.

These words and their meanings will help you enjoy your yoga adventures with Poppy even more! Keep practicing and having fun.

- Yoga: Fun exercises to stretch and move your body.
- Pose: Different ways to stand, sit, or move during yoga.
- Breath: The air you breathe in and out.
- Stretch: Reach out your arms and legs.
- Balance: Stand still without wobbling.
- Quiet Time: Relax and be calm.
- Tree Pose: Stand on one leg like a tree.
- Cat Pose: Pretend to be a soft and stretchy cat.
- Cow Pose: Pretend to be a gentle cow.
- Butterfly Pose: Sit with your feet together and flutter your knees.
- Child's Pose: Sit on your heels, stretch your arms, and rest your head.
- Sun Salutation: A series of stretches to say hello to the day.
- Namaste: A special word for hello and goodbye.
- Mat: A soft surface for yoga.
- Om (Aum): A peaceful sound to say.
- Meditation: Sitting quietly and thinking happy thoughts.
- Inhale: Take a big breath in.
- Exhale: Blow your breath out slowly.
- Focus: Pay attention.
- Relax: Be calm and not worried.

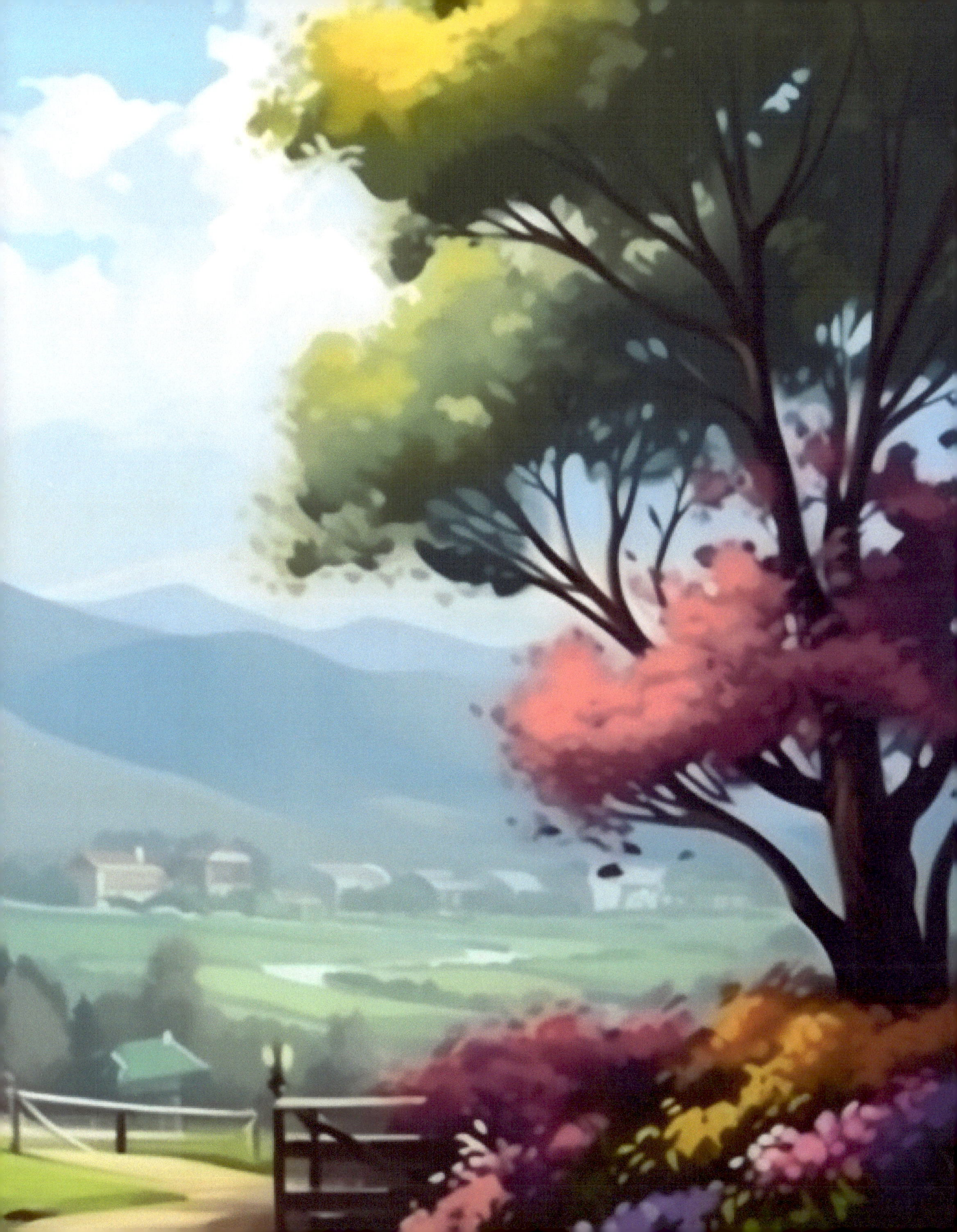

The Furry Friend Series

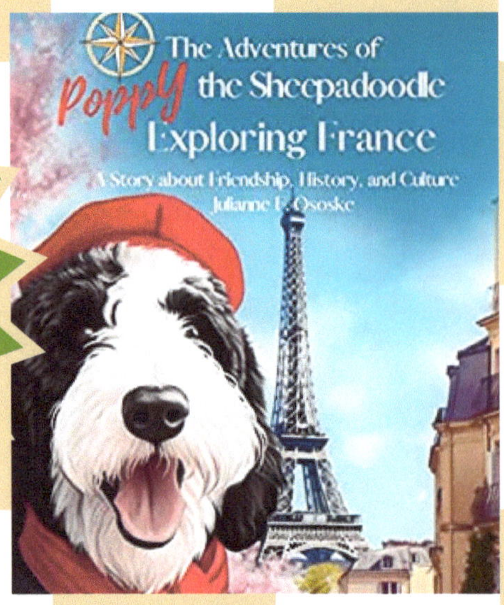

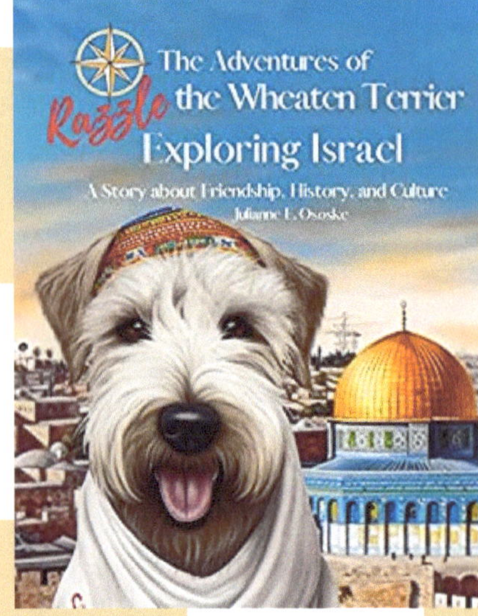

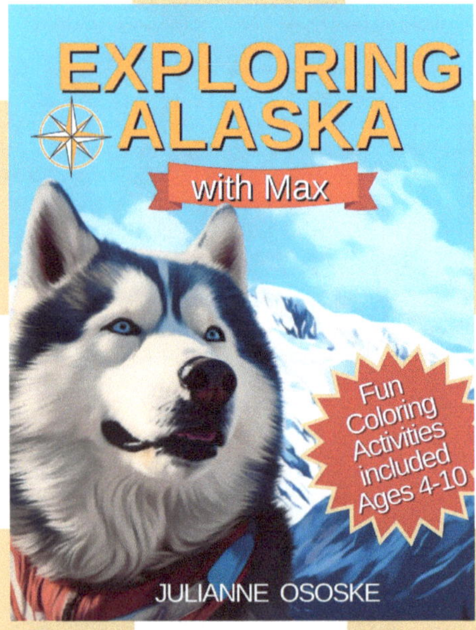

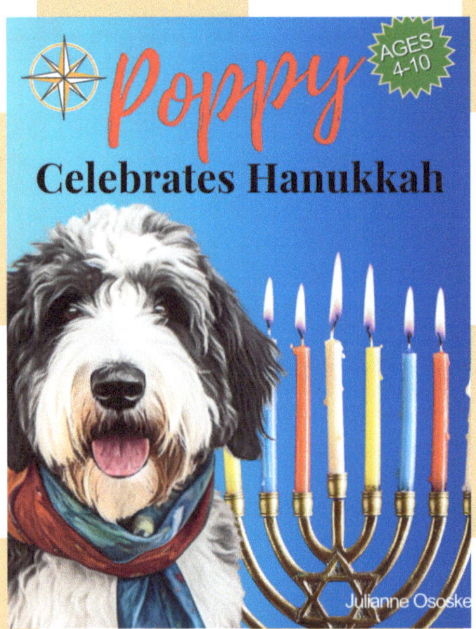

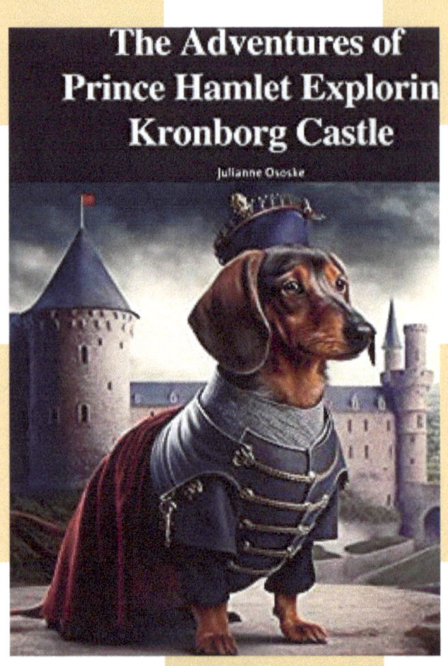

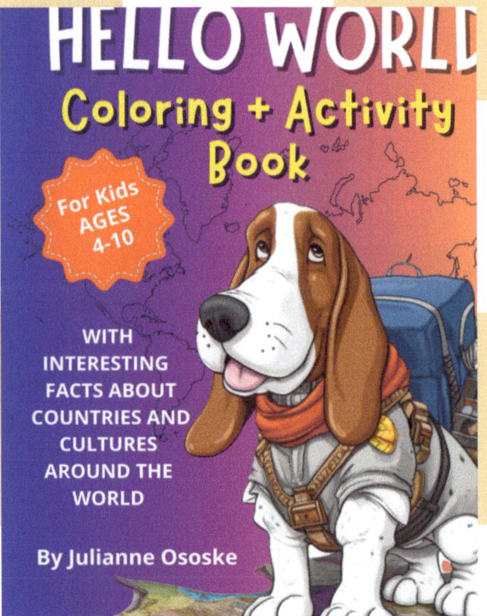

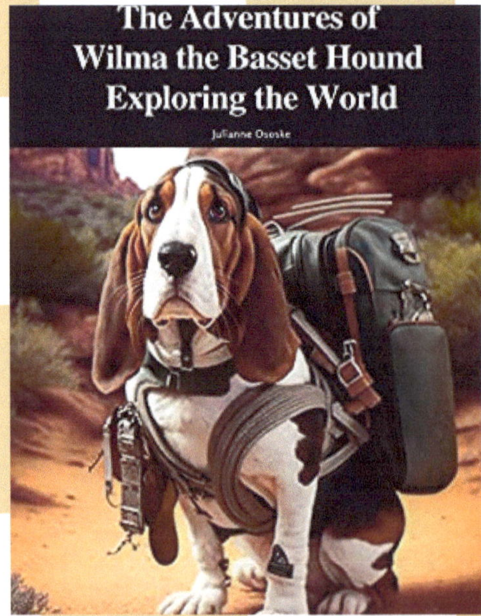

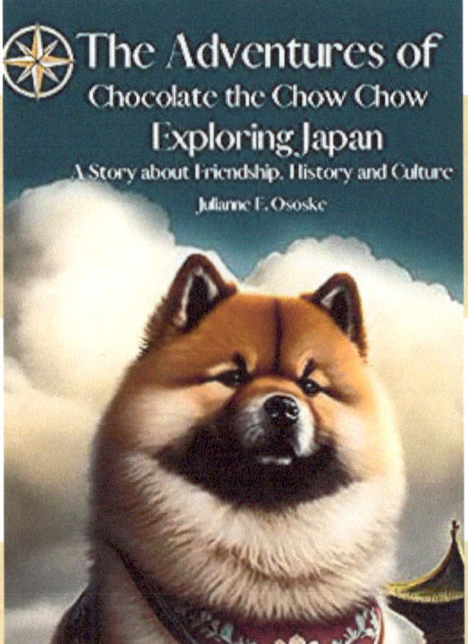

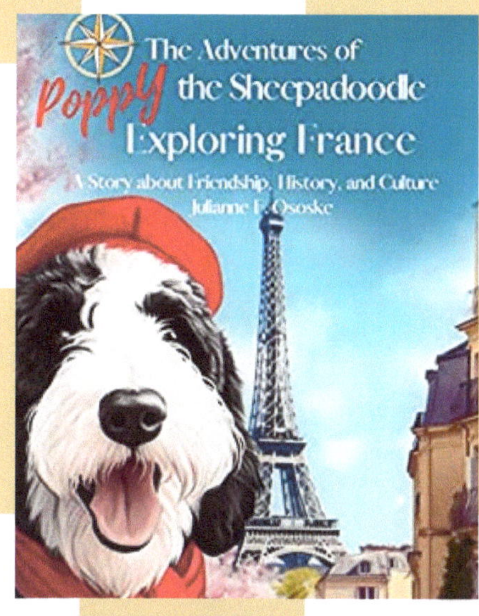

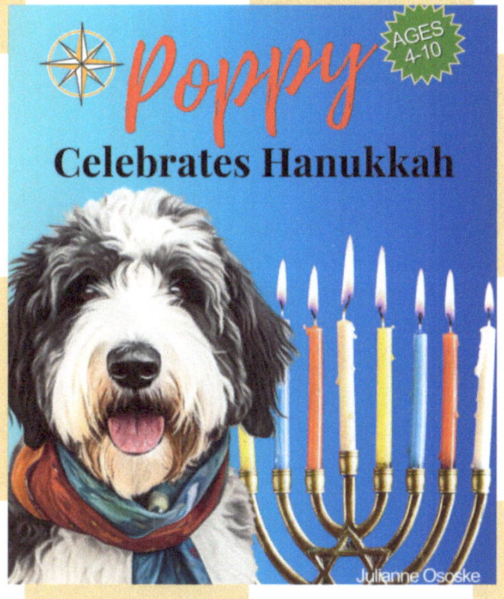

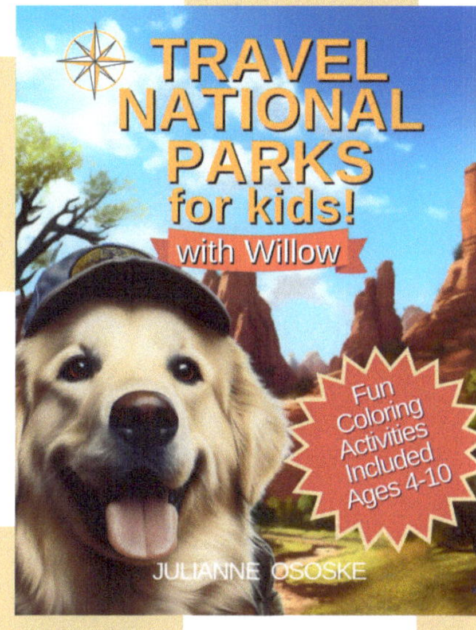

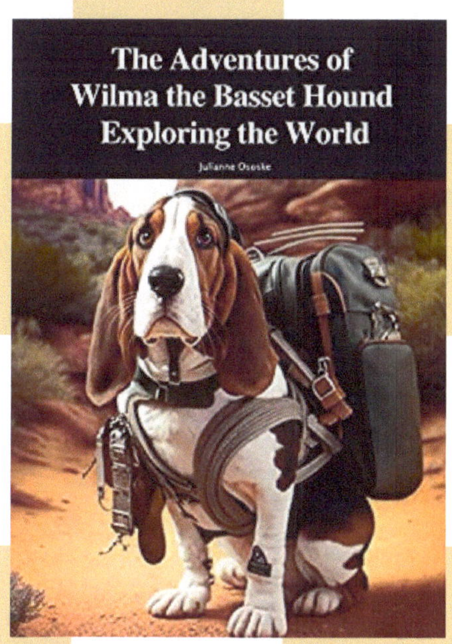

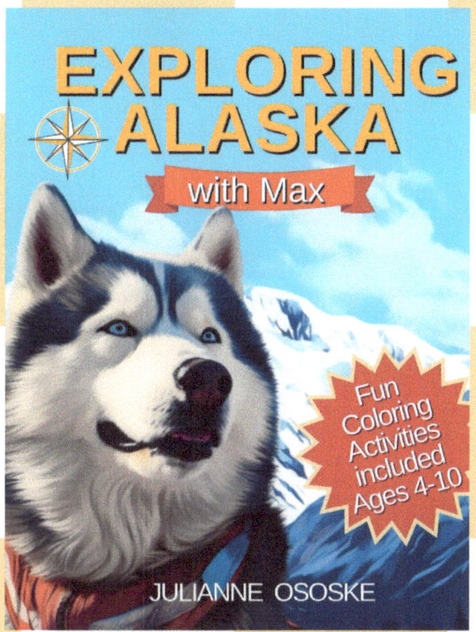

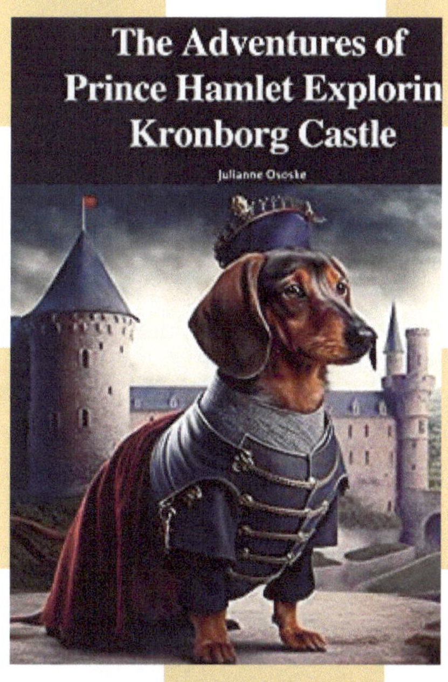

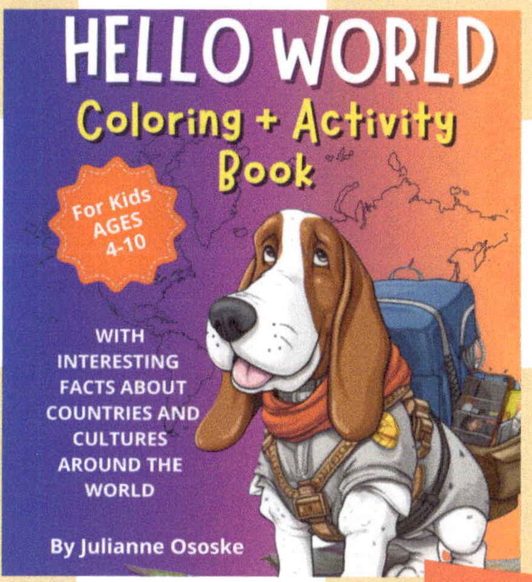

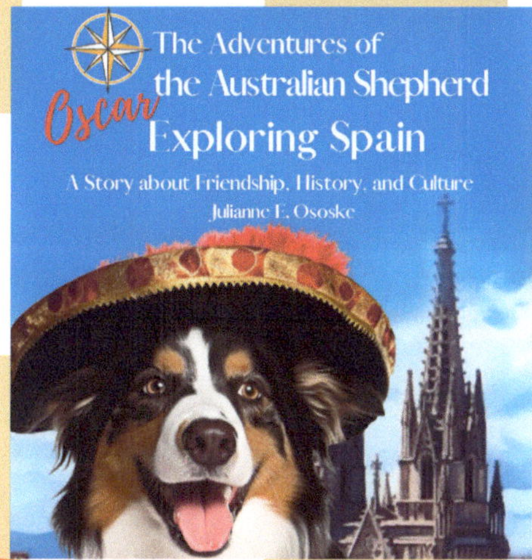

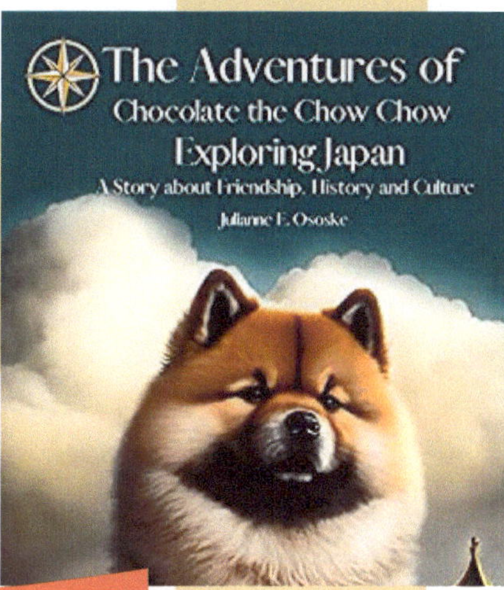

www.OsoskePress.com